The Complete

Lean and Green

Cookbook for Beginners

2022

Quick and easy Lean and Green recipes to Reach Your Greatest Shape and Keep Healthy through the power of "Fueling Hacks Meals".
5 & 1 and 4 & 2 & 1 Meal Plan Included!

Grace Morgan

© Copyright 2022 by Grace Morgan - All rights reserved.

The following Book is reproduced below with the goal of providing information that is as accurate and reliable as possible. Regardless, purchasing this Book can be seen as consent to the fact that both the publisher and the author of this book are in no way experts on the topics discussed within and that any recommendations or suggestions that are made herein are for entertainment purposes only. Professionals should be consulted as needed prior to undertaking any of the action endorsed herein.

This declaration is deemed fair and valid by both the American Bar Association and the Committee of Publishers Association and is legally binding throughout the United States.

Furthermore, the transmission, duplication, or reproduction of any of the following work including specific information will be considered an illegal act irrespective of if it is done electronically or in print. This extends to creating a secondary or tertiary copy of the work or a recorded copy and is only allowed with the express written consent from the Publisher. All additional right reserved.

The information in the following pages is broadly considered a truthful and accurate account of facts and as such, any inattention, use, or misuse of the information in question by the reader will render any resulting actions solely under their purview. There are no scenarios in which the publisher or the original author of this work can be in any fashion deemed liable for any hardship or damages that may befall them after undertaking information described herein.

Additionally, the information in the following pages is intended only for informational purposes and should thus be thought of as universal. As befitting its nature, it is presented without assurance regarding its prolonged validity or interim quality. Trademarks that are mentioned are done without written consent and can in no way be considered an

endorsement from the trademark holder.

Table of Contents

Introduction	5
What is the Lean and Green Diet, and how does it work?	5
What you can eat on the Lean and Green diet:	5
What not to eat on Lean and Green Diet:	6
Benefits of Lean and Green Diet:	6
Tips and Hacks:	6
Fueling Hacks	7
Toasted Almonds	8
Iced Mint Tea	8
Breakfast Shake	9
Energetic Orange Shake	9
Breakfast Porridge	10
The Perfect Hot Chocolate	10
The Happy Hour Punch	11
The Detox Ginger Drink	11
Amazing Strawberry Juice	12
Fresh Fruits Smoothie	12
Lemon Drink	13
Fresh Ginger Smoothie	13
Pumpink Latte	14
Ginger Tea Drink	14
Light Nut and Maple Butter	15
Fabulous Cherry Cider	15
Cranberry Drink	16
Fruits Shake	16
Oatmeal and Carrot Cake	17
Tasty Muffins	17
Breakfast Omelette	18
The Perfect Quinoa	18
Hot Brownies	19
Blueberry Pancakes	19
Sweet Quinoa	20
Honey and Nuts Breakfast	20
Fresh Mango Puree	21
Berries Bowl	21
Fruit Salad	22
Classic Peanut Butter and Jam Bread	22
Pineapple and Spinach Smoothie	23
Energetic Ginger Drink	23
Cabbage and Avocado Smoothie	24
Summer Blueberry and Coconut Ice Cream	25
Spinach and Mango Smoothie	25
Cinnamon Porridge	26
Healthy Chocolate Mousse	26
The Perfect Avocado Dessert	27
"That" Breakfast Porridge	27
Spinach Sauce	28
Shrimp Cocktail	28
Chocolate Mousse	29
Quick Crunchy Toast	29
Quick Cookies Snack	30
Caramel Penuche	30
Chocolate Chia Pudding	31
Tasty Chocolate Custard	31
Apples and Almonds Porridge	32
Fresh and Quick Vanilla Ice Cream	32
Greek-style fruit compote (Hosafi)	33
Vanilla Protein Shake	33
Homemade Breakfast Cereals	34
Strawberry Smoothie	34
Sweet Snack Pudding	35
Cheesecake with Blueberries	35
Carrot Cake	36
Spicy Coffee	36
The Perfect Cereal Breakfast	37
Lunch Recipes	38
Greek Salad	39
Classic Avocado Toast	39
Savory Muffins	40
Delicious Sweet Sandwiches	40
Veggie Risotto	41
Simple Italian Style Risotto	41
The Curious Coconut Soup	42
The Spinach Soup	42
Vegetables Soup	43
Autumn Pumpkin Soup	43
Broccoli Salad	44
Avocado Soup	44
Modern Pasta	45
Orzo Salad	45
Black Bean	46
Sandwiches	46
Cucumber Little Bites	47
Special Cannellini Beans Recipe	47
Quinoa Mix	48
Spicy Hummus	48
Curry Chickpeas	49
French Omelette	49
The Perfect Mushrooms Side Dish	50
Italian Farro	50
Delicious Sweet Bread	51
Special Toast	51
Tasty Risotto	52
Crunchy Asparagus	53
Delicious Tofu	53

Yummy Kale Chips	54
Light Baked Fries	54
Millet and Mix	55
Squash Soup	55
Hot Wrap	56
Summer Pizza	56
Pesto Pita	57
Healthy Turkey Pasta	57
Potato Latke	58
Brussels and Blueberry Salad	58
Everygreen Pumpkin Seed Granola	59
Quick Broccoli Rabe	59
Avocado Quinoa Salad	60
Delicious Whipped Potatoes	60
Delicious Potatoes and Turnips	61
Quick Cauliflower Salad	61
Raw Zoodles	62
Cod Stew with Rice	62
Pinwheels of Feta Cheese and Spinach	63
Sandwich with Artichoke and White Beans	63
Protein Chicken with Rice and Tomato	64
Green Olives Toasted Bread	64
Omelet with Broccoli	65
Couscous with Olives and Beans	65
Roasted Tomatoes with Parmesan	66
Roasted Vegetables	66
Green Soup	67
Roasted Peppers	67
Light Asparagus	68
Corn Peppers Salad	68
Baked Mediterranean Salmon	69
Tuna Salad	69
Beans Salad	70
Dinner Recipes	71
Classic Tofu Stew	72
Classic Hummus	72
Mexican Style Omelette	73
Traditional Spanish Tortilla	73
The Simplest Tahini Sauce	74
Tasty Tapenade	74
Caprese Toast	75
Rainbow Chard Recipe	75
Greek Tahini Sauce	76
Pork Chops	76
Simple Salmon Soup	77
Marinade for Every Dish	77
Bulgur with Spinach and Tomatoes	78
Mussel Stew	78
Chicken Meatballs	79
Patties Kale Salad	79
Quick Pinto Bean Soup with Herbs	80

Hummus of Cauliflower and Avocado	80
Delicious Crispy Sweet Potatoes	81
Carrot Fake Meatballs	81
Garlic Croutons	82
Glazed Carrots – Side Dish	82
Beans Dressing	83
Quick Zucchini Rolls	83
Healthy Zucchini Rolls	84
Roasted Chickpea Snack	84
Seafood Soup	85
Hummus with Tomatoes	85
Tuna Salad with Capers	86
Salad in a Jar	86
Green Beans and Ground Beef	87
Easy Tuna Zoodle Salad	87
Mushroom Cauliflower Risotto	88
Bacon Cheeseburger Wraps	88
Salmon with Chives and Scrambled Eggs	89
Italian Style Omelette	89
Paprika Chicken with Rutabaga	90
Smoked Salmon with Avocado	90
Seeds Crackers	91
Ginger Lime Chicken	91
Stuffed Mozzarella and Basil Meatballs	92
Easy Hot Dog	92
Ham Quiche	93
Cheesy Eggs	93
Tapas	94
Scrambled Feta	94
Healthy Guacamole	95
Pesto Eggs Muffins	95
Mexican Scrambled Eggs	96
Delicious Roasted Chicken	96
Savoury Oven Pancakes	97
Tasty Pork with Fake Fried Eggs	97
Lemon Salmon	98
Rollups with Cheese	98
Corn Fritters	99
Glazed Chicken Wings	99
Cheese Omelet	100
Cheese Waffles	100
Green Creamed Cabbage	101
Bacon Mushrooms Dinner	101
Tortilla Chips	102
Walnut and Zucchini Salad	102
Tasty Briam	103
Indian Crepe	103
The Easiest Polenta Recipe	104
Tomato Sauce	104
5&1 MEAL PLAN	105
4&2&1 MRAL PLAN	107
Conclusion	110

Introduction

What is the Lean and Green Diet, and how does it work?

The method used in the Lean and Green Diet works like this: eat several small meals or snacks every day; this leads to a manageable and sustainable weight loss over time, and then change your habits without trying too hard.
It is a diet created specifically to help people lose weight by reducing calories and carbohydrates through portion-controlled meals and snacks.
Snacks, or rather "Fueling" are bars, pre-packaged foods, homemade smoothies that will help you fight hunger and achieve a sense of satiety.

In addition, you will find Meal Plans that are divided as follows:

- 5 &1 Meal Plan: includes five optimal health foods and a balanced Lean and Green Meal each day. Usually, this is the easiest and fastest way to start the Lean and Green diet since it has several benefits.
- Time: by following this plan, you will save the time you spend in the kitchen because you only have to eat one satiating meal. The rest of the meals are Fueling Hacks that are quick and convenient to carry around.
- The calories you take in are significantly reduced, allowing you to lose weight faster.
- 4 & 2 & 1 Meal Plan includes four Fuelings, two lean and green meals, and one snack per day. This plan was created for those who need more calories or flexibility in food choices.

Don't worry! This eating plan will allow you to lose weight anyway, but gradually.
Drastic diets are not helpful because you would immediately go back to your usual diet since they deprive you of foods you crave.
Both food plans are specially designed to follow the Lean and Green diet in the right way; whichever food plan you choose, it will still allow you not to deprive yourself of the foods you like the most, as the recipes contained in this cookbook are very tasty and suitable for everyone.

Preamble: to follow this diet at its best, you can stick to the list below; in the cookbook, you will find a few recipes that deviate slightly from this list, for the simple reason that we believe that to follow a diet at its best, every now and then you need to treat yourself to something different.

What you can eat on the Lean and Green diet:

- Meat: turkey, pork chop, lean beef, lamb, chicken, tenderloin, ground beef (at least 85% lean)
- Fish and shellfish: trout, salmon, shrimp, halibut, lobster, tuna, crab, scallops
- Eggs: egg whites, whole eggs, egg whisks
- Soy products: tofu
- Vegetable oils: flaxseed, cocoa, walnuts, canola, and olive oil
- Other healthy fats: avocados, olives, almonds, reduced-fat margarine, low carb salad dressings, walnuts, pistachios,
- Low-carb vegetables: spinach, bell peppers, celery, kohlrabi, cucumbers, cabbage, mushrooms, cauliflower, eggplant, broccoli, zucchini, spaghetti squash, jicama
- Sugar-free snacks: chewing gum, jelly, popsicles, mints
- Sugar-free drinks: water, tea, unsweetened almond milk, coffee
- Condiments and seasonings: spices, salt, yellow mustard, 1/2 teaspoon only ketchup, lemon juice, dried herbs, lime juice, soy sauce, sugar-free syrup, salsa, zero-calorie sweeteners, cocktail sauce, or barbecue sauce

❧ What not to eat on Lean and Green Diet:

- Fried foods
- Refined grains: pasta, cookies, white bread, crackers, flour tortillas, white rice, pastries
- Some fats: butter, solid fat
- Whole dairy products: milk, cheese, yogurt
- Alcohol: all varieties
- Sugary drinks: soda, fruit juices, energy drinks, sweet tea

❧ Benefits of Lean and Green Diet:

This diet is ideal for those who can not follow a strict diet. It is pretty easy to follow, and if it is respected, it allows you to see results from the first weeks.

Generally, the average caloric intake of an adult ranges from 1500 to 3000 kcal per day. This diet will be decreased to about 900 kcal per day. And it is precisely this reason why the Lean and Green diet will allow you to burn fat quickly.

In addition, this diet contains an adequate amount of sugar; studies have shown that when a person "detoxes" from too much sugar intake in the past, they begin to feel more energetic and motivated.

❧ Tips and Hacks:

In addition to food plans explicitly designed to reduce calories and therefore lose weight, below you'll find tips and tricks to best build your new healthy lifestyle.

- Drink 2 glasses of water as soon as you wake up on an empty stomach: it improves the health of your hair, is good for your skin, helps you lose weight, gives you energy, and boosts your metabolism.
- Always eat breakfast: it helps regulate your metabolism and makes you feel fuller throughout the day.
- Don't drink alcohol.
- Exercise at least 2/3 times a week; even a brisk walk is good. Also, if you have the chance, you can exercise outdoors, especially when it's cold. According to researchers, cold weather forces our bodies to burn more calories to maintain a constant body temperature.
- Drink 2 liters of water a day. Water cleanses your body of toxins and excess fluids, turning them into waste then expelled.
- Sleep at least 8 hours a night: several studies have shown that sleeping 8 hours helps concentration, productivity, and even weight loss because it affects hormonal and metabolic regulation. Not only that: adequate sleep also affects motivation, hypersensitivity, headaches.
- Sleep on the left side if you can: the stomach and gastric juices remain lower than the esophagus, reducing heartburn and digestive disorders.

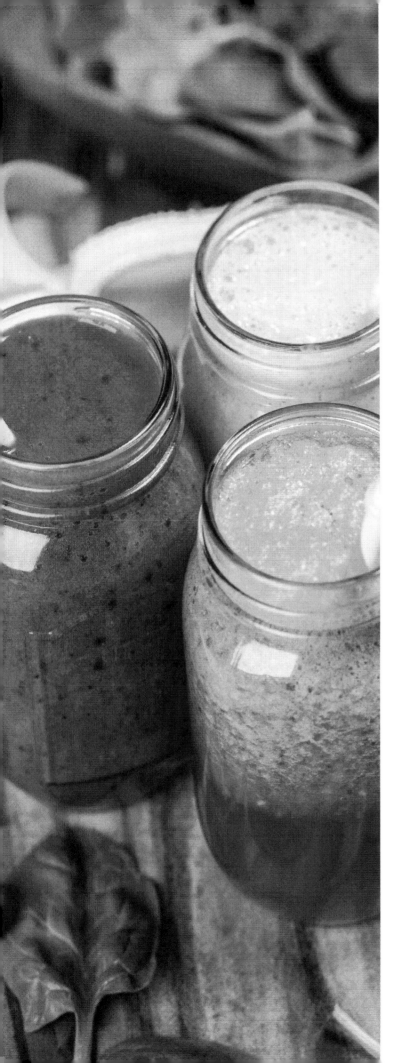

FUELING HACKS MEALS

ICED MINT TEA

COOKING: 0 min **PREPARATION: 5 min** **SERVES: 10**

INGREDIENTS

- 10 cups cold water
- flavorings fresh mint
- 5 cups ice cubes
- 5 tea bags

DIRECTIONS

Leave a pitcher full of water in the refrigerator for 1-2 hours.
Combine the tea bags, fresh mint, and half of the cold water.
Remove the tea bag and flavoring.
Add the ice cubes, the rest of the cold water and serve.

NUTRITION:

Per Serving: Calories 0 | Protein 0 | Carbs 0

TOASTED ALMONDS

COOKING: 10 min **PREPARATION: 2 min** **SERVES: 1**

INGREDIENTS

- ½ cup raw almonds or sunflower seeds
- 2 tablespoons tamari or soy sauce
- 1 teaspoon toasted sesame oil

DIRECTIONS

Prepare the ingredients.
Heat a skillet over medium heat, then add the almonds, often stirring to prevent burning.
Once the almonds are toasted, about 8 minutes for the almonds or 5 minutes for the sunflower seeds, pour the sesame oil and tamari into the hot pan and stir well.
Turn off the heat, and as the almonds cool, the tamari mixture will stick and dry on the nuts.

NUTRITION:

Per Serving: Calories 89 | Protein 4g | Carbohydrates 3g

ENERGETIC ORANGE SHAKE

COOKING: 0 min **PREPARATION: 5 min** **SERVES: 2**

INGREDIENTS

- 1 orange, peeled
- ¼ cup vegan yogurt
- 2 tbsp. orange juice
- ¼ tsp vanilla extract
- 4 ice cubes

DIRECTIONS

Place the vanilla extract, vegan yogurt, orange, ice cubes, and orange juice in a blender. Blend all ingredients well until smooth and well combined.
Pour into smoothie glasses and serve.

NUTRITION:
Per Serving: Calories 120 | Protein 10g | Carbohydrates 23g

BREAKFAST SHAKE

COOKING: 0 min **PREPARATION: 3-5 min** **SERVES: 2**

INGREDIENTS

- 3 tablespoons, raw cacao powder
- 1 cup, almond milk
- 2 frozen bananas
- 3 tablespoons, natural peanut butter

DIRECTIONS

Use a powerful blender to combine all the ingredients and blend until smooth and homogeneous.
Enjoy a hearty smoothie to kick-start your day.

NUTRITION:
Per Serving: Calories 150 | Protein 11g | Carbohydrates 41g

THE PERFECT HOT CHOCOLATE

COOKING: 5 min **PREPARATION:** 3 min **SERVES:** 4

INGREDIENTS

- 1/3 cup of cocoa powder, unsweetened
- 1/3 cup of coconut sugar
- 1/8 teaspoon of salt
- 1/8 teaspoon of ground cinnamon
- 1 teaspoon of vanilla extract, unsweetened
- 32 fluid ounce of coconut milk

DIRECTIONS

In a saucepan, add all the ingredients and mix well.
Turn on the heat over low heat, and stir until the chocolate has thickened.

NUTRITION:

Per Serving: Calories 67 | Protein 2g | Carbohydrates 13g

BREAKFAST PORRIDGE

COOKING: 25 min **PREPARATION:** 10 min **SERVES:** 8

INGREDIENTS

- 2 cup amaranth
- 2 cinnamon sticks
- 4 bananas, diced
- 2 Tbsp chopped pecans
- 4 cups water

DIRECTIONS

In a saucepan, combine the banana, cinnamon sticks, water and amaranth.
Cover and let simmer for about 20 minutes.
Remove from heat and discard cinnamon. Arrange in bowls and top with pecans.

NUTRITION:

Per Serving: Calories 270 | Protein 10g | Carbohydrates 54g

THE DETOX GINGER DRINK

COOKING: 5 min **PREPARATION: 10 min** **SERVES: 2**

INGREDIENTS

- 1/2 teaspoon of grated ginger, fresh
- 1 small lemon slice
- 1/8 teaspoon of cayenne pepper
- 1/8 teaspoon of ground turmeric
- 1/8 teaspoon of ground cinnamon
- 1 teaspoon of maple syrup
- 1 teaspoon of apple cider vinegar
- 2 cups of boiling water

DIRECTIONS

Pour the boiling water into a small saucepan, add and stir the ginger, and rest for 8 to 10 minutes before covering the pan. Pass the mixture through a strainer and into the liquid, add the cayenne pepper, turmeric, cinnamon, and stir properly. Add the maple syrup, vinegar, and lemon slice.
Add and stir an infused lemon and serve immediately.

NUTRITION:
Per Serving: Calories 32 | Protein 10g | Carbohydrates 0

THE HAPPY HOUR PUNCH

COOKING: 3h **PREPARATION: 10 min** **SERVES: 10**

INGREDIENTS

- 3 cinnamon sticks, each about 3 inches long
- 12 whole cloves
- 1/2 cup of coconut sugar
- 1/3 cup of lemon juice
- 32 fluid ounce of pomegranate juice
- 32 fluid ounce of apple juice, unsweetened
- 16 fluid ounces of brewed tea

DIRECTIONS

Using a 4-quart slow cooker, pour the lemon juice, pomegranate, apple juice, tea, and sugar.
Wrap the whole cloves and cinnamon stick in a cheesecloth, tie its corners with a string, and immerse it in the liquid present in the slow cooker.
Then cover it with the lid, plug in the slow cooker and let it cook at the low heat setting for 3 hours or until heated thoroughly.
When done, discard the cheesecloth bag and serve it hot or cold.

NUTRITION:
Per Serving: Calories 240 | Protein 7g | Carbohydrates 58g

FRESH FRUITS SMOOTHIE

COOKING: 0 min | **PREPARATION: 10 min** | **SERVES: 1**

INGREDIENTS

- ¾ cup soy yogurt
- ½ cup pineapple juice
- 1 cup pineapple chunks
- 1 cup raspberries, sliced
- 1 cup blueberries, sliced

DIRECTIONS

Process the ingredients in a blender.
Chill before serving.

NUTRITION:
Per Serving: Calories 279 | Protein 12g | Carbohydrates 36g

AMAZING STRAWBERRY JUICE

COOKING: 1 min | **PREPARATION: 5 min** | **SERVES: 6**

INGREDIENTS

- 2 cup strawberries
- 1 cup sugar or as per taste
- 7 cups of water
- 2 cup lemon juice
- Sliced berries for garnish

DIRECTIONS

Combine the water and sugar in a bowl and microwave it without melting it completely. Add the strawberries and 1 cup of water in a blender and blend.

Combine the strawberry puree with the water dissolved in the sugar and mix.

Pour in the lime juice and water if needed. Mix well and chill before serving. You can add berries on top as a garnish.

NUTRITION:
Per Serving: Calories 144 | Protein 37g | Carbohydrates 29g

FRESH GINGER SMOOTHIE

COOKING: 0 min | **PREPARATION: 5 min** | **SERVES: 2**

INGREDIENTS

- 1 banana
- ½ apple sliced
- 1 orange sliced and peeled
- 1 lemon juice
- 2 big spinach
- 1 tbsp. fresh ginger
- ½ cup almond milk

DIRECTIONS

Grab a blender. Peel and slice all the fruit. Add and blend the ginger, orange, banana, apple, lime juice, and spinach.
Now add the almond milk and pulse for a few more seconds. You can add chia seeds, apples, or raspberries for a bowl of smoothies. Store for up to 10 hours in the refrigerator.

NUTRITION:
Per Serving: Calories 130 | Protein 10g | Carbohydrates 32g

LEMON DRINK

COOKING: 2h | **PREPARATION: 10 min** | **SERVES: 2**

INGREDIENTS

- 1 cinnamon stick, about 3 inches long
- 1/2 teaspoon of whole cloves
- 2 cups of coconut sugar
- 4 fluid of ounce pineapple juice
- 1/2 cup and 2 tablespoons of lemon juice
- 12 fluid ounces of orange juice
- 2 1/2 quarts of water

DIRECTIONS

Pour water into a 6-quarts slow cooker and stir the sugar and lemon juice properly.
Wrap the cinnamon with the whole cloves in cheesecloth and tie its corners with string.
Immerse this cheesecloth bag in the liquid present in the slow cooker and cover it with the lid.
Then plug in the slow cooker and let it cook on a high heat setting for 2 hours or until heated thoroughly. When done, discard the cheesecloth bag and serve the drink hot or cold.

NUTRITION:
Per Serving: Calories 15 | Protein 1g | Carbohydrates 3.2g

GINGER TEA DRINK

COOKING: 2h   **PREPARATION: 10 min**   **SERVES: 6**

INGREDIENTS

- 1 tablespoon of minced ginger root
- 2 tablespoons of honey
- 15 green tea bags
- 32 fluid ounce of white grape juice
- 2 quarts of boiling water

DIRECTIONS

Pour water into a 4-quarts slow cooker, immerse tea bags, cover the cooker and let stand for 10 minutes.

After 10 minutes, remove and discard tea bags and stir in the remaining ingredients.

Return cover to slow cooker, then plugin and let cook at high heat setting for 2 hours or until heated through. When done, strain the liquid and serve hot or cold.

NUTRITION:

Per Serving: Calories 45 | Protein 2g | Carbohydrates 12g

PUMPINK LATTE

COOKING: 0 min   **PREPARATION: 5 min**   **SERVES: 4**

INGREDIENTS

- 2 tsp pumpkin pie spice or ground ginger
- 2 pinches vanilla extract
- 4 tbsp maple syrup
- 3 cups coffee
- 4 cups milk

DIRECTIONS

In a small saucepan, add the milk, maple syrup, coffee and spices.

Stir until it boils.

Pour pumpkin spice milk through a strainer and serve.

NUTRITION:

Per Serving: Calories 112 | Protein 9g | Carbs 20g

FABULOUS CHERRY CIDER

COOKING: 3h | **PREPARATION: 10 min** | **SERVES: 12**

INGREDIENTS

- 2 cinnamon sticks, each about 3 inches long
- 6-ounce of cherry gelatin
- 4 quarts of apple cider

DIRECTIONS

Using a 6-quarts slow cooker, pour the apple cider and add the cinnamon stick.

Stir, then cover the slow cooker with its lid. Plugin the cooker and let it cook for 3 hours at the high heat setting or until heated thoroughly.

Then add and stir the gelatin properly, then continue cooking for another hour.

When done, remove the cinnamon sticks and serve the drink hot or cold.

NUTRITION:
Per Serving: Calories 99 | Protein 0.3g | Carbohydrates 2g

LIGHT NUT AND MAPLE BUTTER

COOKING: 0 min | **PREPARATION: 20 min** | **SERVES: 2**

INGREDIENTS

- ½ tablespoon ground flaxseed
- 1 teaspoon ground cinnamon
- ½ tablespoon maple syrup
- 2 tablespoons cashew milk
- ¾ cups crunchy, unsweetened peanut butter

DIRECTIONS

Combine cashew milk, cinnamon, flax seeds, maple syrup, and peanut butter.

Mix everything together as if you were scrambling eggs.

If it's too runny, add a bit more peanut butter.

If it's too thick, add a bit of cashew milk.

Add foil on top and refrigerate for about 30 minutes. Serve!

NUTRITION:
Per Serving: Calories 201 | Protein 21g | Carbohydrates 29g

FRUITS SHAKE

COOKING: 0 min **PREPARATION: 5 min** **SERVES: 2**

INGREDIENTS

- 1 cup oatmeal, already prepared, cooled
- 1 apple, cored, roughly chopped
- 1 banana, halved
- 1 cup baby spinach
- 2 cups coconut water
- 2 cups ice, cubed
- ½ tsp ground cinnamon
- 1 tsp pure vanilla extract

DIRECTIONS

Add all ingredients to a blender.
Blend until smooth and homogeneous.
Taste.

NUTRITION:
Per Serving: Calories 170 | Protein 5g | Carbohydrates 15g

CRANBERRY DRINK

COOKING: 3h **PREPARATION: 10 min** **SERVES: 12**

INGREDIENTS

- 1 1/2 cups of coconut sugar
- 12 whole cloves
- 2 fluid ounces of lemon juice
- 6 fluid ounces of orange juice
- 32 fluid ounces of cranberry juice
- 8 cups of hot water
- 1/2 cup of Red Hot candies

DIRECTIONS

Pour the water into a 6-quarts slow cooker, cranberry juice, orange juice, and lemon juice.
Stir the sugar properly.
Wrap the whole cloves in a cheesecloth, tie its corners with strings, and immerse it in the liquid present inside the slow cooker.
Add the red hot candies to the slow cooker and cover it with the lid.
Then plug in the slow cooker and let it cook on the low heat setting for 3 hours or until heated thoroughly.
When done, discard the cheesecloth bag and serve.

NUTRITION:
Per Serving: Calories 89; Protein 0g; Carbohydrates 0g

TASTY MUFFINS

COOKING: 10 min   **PREPARATION: 10 min**   **SERVES: 10**

INGREDIENTS

- ½ cup hot water
- ½ cup raisins
- ¼ cup ground flax seeds
- 2 cups rolled oats
- ¼ teaspoon sea salt
- ½ cup walnuts
- ¼ teaspoon baking soda
- 1 banana
- 2 tablespoons cinnamon
- ¼ cup maple syrup

DIRECTIONS

Whisk flax seeds with water and let the mixture sit for about 5 minutes.
In a food processor, blend all ingredients together with the flaxseed blend.
Blend everything for 20 seconds, but do not create a substance.
Place the made batter mixture into cupcake molds and place it on a baking sheet.
You will need cupcake liners. Bake everything for about 25 minutes at 350 degrees.
Enjoy the freshly made cookies with a glass of warm milk.

NUTRITION:
Per Serving: Calories 133| Protein 3g| Carbohydrates 27g

OATMEAL AND CARROT CAKE

COOKING: 15 min   **PREPARATION: 10 min**   **SERVES: 2**

INGREDIENTS

- 1 cup water
- ½ teaspoon cinnamon
- 1 cup, rolled oats
- Salt
- ¼ cup, raisins
- ½ cup, shredded carrots
- 1 cup, non-dairy milk
- ¼ teaspoon, allspice
- ½ teaspoon, vanilla extract
- Toppings:
- ¼ cup, chopped walnuts
- 2 tablespoons, maple syrup
- 2 tablespoons, shredded coconut

DIRECTIONS

Place a small saucepan over low heat and bring the non-dairy milk, oats, and water to a boil.
Add the raisins, cinnamon, carrots, salt, vanilla extract, and allspice and stir. You'll know they're ready when the liquid is fully absorbed into all the ingredients (in about 10 minutes).
Transfer the thickened dish to bowls. You can garnish with maple syrup on top with coconut or nuts.

NUTRITION:
Per Serving: Calories 110 | Protein 4g | Carbohydrates 10g

THE PERFECT QUINOA

COOKING: 20 min   **PREPARATION: 10 min**   **SERVES: 6**

INGREDIENTS

- 1 ½ teaspoons vanilla extract
- 3 tablespoons honey
- 3 pitted, finely chopped dried dates
- ⅓ cup and 2 teaspoons milk
- 1 ½ teaspoons sea salt
- 7 ½ finely chopped dried apricots
- ⅓ cup and 2 teaspoons chopped raw almonds
- 1 ½ teaspoon ground cinnamon
- 1 ½ cups quinoa

DIRECTIONS

1. In a skillet, toast almonds over medium heat until just golden brown, about 5 minutes; set aside.
2. In a saucepan, add the quinoa and cinnamon together over medium heat until heated through.
3. Add the milk and sea salt to the saucepan and stir; bring the mixture to a boil, lower the heat, place a lid on the saucepan, and let simmer for 10 minutes.
4. Stir the dates, honey, vanilla, apricots, and half of the almonds into the quinoa mixture. Add the remaining almonds to serve.

NUTRITION:

Per Serving: Calories 328 | Protein 10g | Carbohydrates 41g

BREAKFAST OMELETTE

COOKING: 10 min   **PREPARATION: 5 min**   **SERVES: 4**

INGREDIENTS

- ⅔ (10 ounces) package of fresh spinach
- 8 large eggs, lightly beaten
- salt and ground black pepper to taste
- ¼ cup cream cheese, cut into small pieces
- 2 tablespoons and 2 teaspoons butter
- ⅔ cup mushrooms, sliced
- 2 ⅔ cloves garlic, minced

DIRECTIONS

Melt butter in a large skillet over medium heat; add garlic and mushrooms and cook until garlic is fragrant, about 1 minute. Add the spinach and cook until the spinach is wilted for about 4 minutes.
Add and stir in the eggs; season with salt and pepper.
Cook, without stirring, until eggs begin to firm; turn.
Sprinkle cream cheese over the egg mixture and bake until cream cheese begins to soften about 5 minutes.

NUTRITION:

Per Serving: Calories 268 | Protein 11g | Carbohydrates 6g

BLUEBERRY PANCAKES

COOKING: 10 min | **PREPARATION: 5 min** | **SERVES: 4**

INGREDIENTS

- 6 eggs
- 3 oz. fresh blueberries
- ½ cup cream cheese
- 2/3 cup almond flour
- 2/3 cup oat fiber
- ½ lemon, the zest
- 3 oz. Coconut oil
- 2 tsp baking powder

DIRECTIONS

Mix eggs, coconut oil, and cream cheese in a bowl.
Combine the rest of the ingredients separately, except the blueberries.
Once ready, pour into the egg mixture.
Mix very well until a smooth batter is obtained and let stand for 5-7 minutes.
In a skillet over medium heat, fry the pancakes.
Use for each pancake about ⅓ cup of mixture.
Let fry for 2-3 minutes, and then add blueberries.
Flip pancakes and fry for a few more minutes.

NUTRITION:
Per Serving: Calories 208 | Protein 12g | Carbs 32g

HOT BROWNIES

COOKING: 25 min | **PREPARATION: 10 min** | **SERVES: 12**

INGREDIENTS

- 1½ eggs
- 2/5 cup erythritol
- 1/6 cup cocoa powder
- ½ oz. dark chocolate with a minimum of 90% cocoa solids
- ½ cup almond flour
- ¼ tsp baking powder
- 1/6 cup almond butter
- 1 tbsp water
- ½ tbsp vanilla extract
- 3 oz. butter softened
- 1/8 tsp salt

DIRECTIONS

Place baking paper on top of a baking sheet and preheat the oven to 350°F (175°C) degrees.
Combine the eggs, sweetener, almond butter, and butter in a bowl. Mix well until the mixture is smooth.
Stir together the almond flour, , salt, cocoa powder, water, baking powder, instant coffee powder, and vanilla extract.
Chop the chocolate bar and add it to the resulting mixture.
In a baking pan, pour the mixture and smooth the surface with a spatula since the batter will be quite thick.
Bake in the oven for about 25 minutes. Be careful not to overcook, be careful, or the bars will be dry.
Allow the brownies to cool before cutting and serving.

NUTRITION:
Per Serving: Calories 108 | Protein 2g | Carbs 22g

SWEET QUINOA

COOKING: 20 min   **PREPARATION: 10 min**   **SERVES: 6**

INGREDIENTS

- ¾ cup chopped almonds
- ½ cup flax seeds
- 1 ½ teaspoon ground cinnamon
- ¾ teaspoon ground nutmeg
- ⅓ cup and 2 teaspoons water
- 1 ½ cups rinsed quinoa
- ¾ cup chopped dried apricots

DIRECTIONS

1. In a saucepan, add water and cook quinoa over medium heat;
2. Bring to a boil and reduce heat and simmer until most of the water has been absorbed for about 10 minutes.
3. Add and stir in almonds, apricots, cinnamon, flaxseed, and nutmeg; cook until quinoa is tender, about 3 minutes.

NUTRITION:

Per Serving: Calories 328 | Protein 9g | Carbohydrates 45g

HONEY AND NUTS BREAKFAST

COOKING: 30 min   **PREPARATION: 10 min**   **SERVES: 6**

INGREDIENTS

- 1 cup brown rice, uncooked
- ½ cup raisins, seedless
- 1 tsp cinnamon, ground
- ¼ Tbsp peanut butter
- 2 ¼ cups water
- Honey, to taste
- Nuts, toasted

DIRECTIONS

In a saucepan, combine the raisins, rice, cinnamon, and butter. Add 2 ¼ cups water and bring to a boil.
Cover the rice and cook over low heat until cooked.
Brush with a fork. Add honey and nuts to taste.

NUTRITION:

Per Serving: Calories 160 | Protein 3g | Carbohydrates 24g

FRESH MANGO PUREE

COOKING: 30 min **PREPARATION: 10 min** **SERVES: 12**

INGREDIENTS

- 6 mangoes
- ½ cup honey
- 1 cup heavy cream

DIRECTIONS

Bring water to a boil in a saucepan, place whole mangoes in and simmer.
Remove the mangoes from the water and let them cool for about 30 minutes.
In a bowl, whisk the honey and cream until frothy.
Remove the skin and pits from the mangoes.
Blend and reduce to a puree.
Add the resulting mango puree to the cream mixture and combine.
Pour into dessert bowls and chill for about 3 hours in the refrigerator.
Serve.

NUTRITION:
Per Serving: Calories 179 | Protein 2g | Carbohydrates 30g

BERRIES BOWL

COOKING: 0 min **PREPARATION: 10 min** **SERVES: 2**

INGREDIENTS

- 1 ½ cups of coconut milk
- 2 small bananas
- 1 cup mixed berries, frozen
- 2 tablespoons almond butter
- 1 tablespoon chia seeds
- 2 tablespoons granola

DIRECTIONS

Add the chia seeds, bananas, almond butter berries, and coconut milk.
Puree until creamy, even, and smooth.
Divide the blended mixture into each bowl and top with granola.
Serve immediately.

NUTRITION:
Per Serving: Calories: 203 | Protein: 6g | Carbohydrates: 33g

FRUIT SALAD

COOKING: 10 min **PREPARATION: 10 min** **SERVES: 4**

INGREDIENTS

- ½ cup fresh lemon juice
- ¼ cup agave syrup
- 1 teaspoon fresh ginger, grated
- ½ teaspoon vanilla extract
- 1 banana, sliced
- 2 cups mixed berries
- 1 cup seedless grapes
- 2 cups apples, cored and diced

DIRECTIONS

In a saucepan, mix the agave syrup, lemon juice, and ginger and bring to a boil over medium heat.

Then, lower the heat and let it simmer for about 5 minutes until thick.

Remove from the heat and stir in the vanilla extract. Allow cooling.

Layer the fruit in serving bowls. Pour the cooled sauce over the fruit and serve it well chilled.

NUTRITION:

Per Serving: Calories: 164 | Protein: 2g | Carbohydrates: 42g

CLASSIC PEANUT BUTTER AND JAM BREAD

COOKING: 10 min **PREPARATION: 5 min** **SERVES: 2**

INGREDIENTS

- 1 cup flour
- 1/2 teaspoon baking powder
- 1/2 teaspoon sea salt
- 1 teaspoon coconut sugar
- 1/2 cup warm water
- 3 teaspoons olive oil
- 3 tablespoons peanut butter
- 3 tablespoons raspberry jam

DIRECTIONS

Mix yeast, flour, sugar, and salt together. Gradually add the water until the dough is uniform.

Divide dough into two balls; flatten each ball to create circles. Heat 1 teaspoon olive oil in a skillet over medium heat. Cook the bread for about 10 minutes or until golden brown.

Serve the bread with peanut butter and raspberry jam. Enjoy!

NUTRITION:

Per Serving: Calories: 293 | Protein: 5| Carbohydrates: 35g

ENERGETIC GINGER DRINK

COOKING: 10 min | **PREPARATION: 5 min** | **SERVES: 2**

INGREDIENTS

- 1/2 teaspoon grated ginger, fresh
- 1 small lemon slice
- 1/8 teaspoon cayenne pepper
- 1/8 teaspoon ground turmeric
- 1/8 teaspoon ground cinnamon
- 1 teaspoon maple syrup
- 1 teaspoon apple cider vinegar
- 2 cups boiling water

DIRECTIONS

In a saucepan, bring the water with the ginger to a boil.
Strain the mixture through a sieve into a bowl.
Add the rest of the ingredients and stir.

NUTRITION:
Per Serving: Calories 80 | Protein 0g | Carbohydrates 0g

PINEAPPLE AND SPINACH SMOOTHIE

COOKING: 0 min | **PREPARATION: 10 min** | **SERVES: 1**

INGREDIENTS

- ½ cup almond milk
- ¼ cup soy yogurt
- 1 cup spinach
- 1 cup banana
- 1 cup pineapple chunks
- 1 tablespoon chia seeds

DIRECTIONS

Add the milk, yogurt, spinach, banana, pineapple, and chia seeds to a blender.
Blend until smooth.
Tip: Let the smoothie rest in the fridge for 15 minutes, then enjoy!

NUTRITION:
Per Serving: Calories 144 | Protein 13g | Carbohydrates 34g

CARROT AND KIWI SMOOTHIE

COOKING: 0 min — **PREPARATION: 5 min** — **SERVES: 2**

INGREDIENTS

- 2 carrots
- 2 kiwis
- fresh mint

DIRECTIONS

Cut the carrots into slices on a cutting board.
Peel the kiwifruit and extract the pulp. Afterward, cut them thinly.
In a blender, add the carrots, kiwis, and mint.
Enjoy the smoothie in a glass with ice!

NUTRITION:

Per Serving: Calories 56 | Protein 4g | Carbohydrates 0g

CABBAGE AND AVOCADO SMOOTHIE

COOKING: 0 min — **PREPARATION: 10 min** — **SERVES: 1**

INGREDIENTS

- 1 ripe banana
- 1 cup of kale
- 1 cup almond milk
- ¼ avocado
- 1 tablespoon chia seeds
- 2 tablespoons honey
- 1 cup ice cubes

DIRECTIONS

Blend the banana, kale, milk, avocado, chia seeds, honey, and ice until smooth.

NUTRITION:

Per Serving: Calories 343 | Protein 6g | Carbohydrates 55g

SPINACH AND MANGO SMOOTHIE

COOKING: 0 min   **PREPARATION: 5 min**   **SERVES: 1**

INGREDIENTS

- 2 cups spinach
- 2 mangoes, ripe, peeled and diced

DIRECTIONS

Bring the water to a boil in a pot. Then, cook the spinach for 15 minutes.

Drain the spinach and add it to a blender along with the mangoes. Then, add the spinach cooking water a little to decide on the consistency.

Blend everything until smooth.

NUTRITION:
Per Serving: Calories: 170 | Protein: 7.2g | Carbohydrates: 102g

SUMMER BLUEBERRY AND COCONUT ICE CREAM

COOKING: 0 min   **PREPARATION: 5 min**   **SERVES: 4**

INGREDIENTS

- 1/4 cup of coconut cream
- 1 tablespoon maple syrup
- ¼ cup coconut flour
- 1 cup blueberries
- ¼ cup blueberries for garnish

DIRECTIONS

Place the coconut cream, maple syrup, coconut flour, blueberries in the food processor and blend everything quickly. Pour the mixture and add the remaining blueberries and mix.

Pour mixture into silicone molds and freeze in the freezer for about 6 hours.

Serve cold and enjoy!

NUTRITION:
Per Serving: Calories 86 | Protein 3g | Carbohydrates 47g

HEALTHY CHOCOLATE MOUSSE

COOKING: 5 min **PREPARATION: 5 min** **SERVES: 2**

INGREDIENTS

- 1/2 cup of coconut milk
- 1 tablespoon maple syrup
- 1-3 tablespoons of cocoa powder
- Pinch of instant coffee
- 2 tbsp. coconut cream
- Blackberries for the garnish

DIRECTIONS

In a saucepan, heat for the coconut milk and maple syrup. When it gets hot, add the coffee and cocoa to the milk mixture.
Remove from the heat and pour into a bowl.
Add the cream to the mixture and whip until firm.
Add some berries and a spoonful of coconut cream.
Enjoy!

NUTRITION:

Per Serving: Calories 162 | Protein 3g | Carbohydrates 13g

CINNAMON PORRIDGE

COOKING: 5 min **PREPARATION: 5 min** **SERVES: 3**

INGREDIENTS

- 3 cups of almond milk
- 3 tablespoons maple syrup
- 3 teaspoons of coconut oil
- 1/4 teaspoon kosher salt
- 1/2 teaspoon ground cinnamon
- 1 ¼ cups semolina

DIRECTIONS

In a saucepan, heat the maple syrup, salt and cinnamon, almond milk and coconut oil over medium heat.
Once hot, gradually add the semolina flour, stirring. Continue to cook until the porridge thickens.
Enjoy!

NUTRITION:

Per Serving: Calories: 321 | Protein: 16g | Carbohydrates: 7g

"THAT" BREAKFAST PORRIDGE

COOKING: 30 min   **PREPARATION: 10 min**   **SERVES: 4**

INGREDIENTS

- 3/4 cup of steel-cut oats, rinsed and soaked overnight
- 3/4 cup of whole barley, rinsed and soaked overnight
- 1/2 cup of cornmeal
- 1 teaspoon of salt
- 3 tablespoons of brown sugar
- 1 cinnamon stick, about 3 inches long
- 1 teaspoon of vanilla extract, unsweetened
- 4 1/2 cups of water

DIRECTIONS

Place all ingredients in a pot and stir well.
Cover the pot and simmer for about 30 minutes, stirring halfway through cooking.
Serve oatmeal with fruit.

NUTRITION:
Per Serving: Calories 129 | Protein 5g | Carbohydrates 22g

THE PERFECT AVOCADO DESSERT

COOKING: 0 min   **PREPARATION: 10 min**   **SERVES: 8**

INGREDIENTS

- 1 cup of milk
- 2 avocados, peeled and pitted
- 1 teaspoon vanilla extract
- 3 teaspoon sweetener

DIRECTIONS

In a food processor, blend the 2 avocados.
Stir in the sweetener, vanilla, and milk until smooth.
Let cool for about 10 minutes before serving.

NUTRITION:
Per Serving: Calories 153 | Protein 12g | Carbohydrates 30g

SHRIMP COCKTAIL

COOKING: 5 min   **PREPARATION:** 5 min   **SERVES:** 6

INGREDIENTS

- ¾ tsp chili flakes
- 3 tbsp coconut oil or ghee
- 3 tbsp finely chopped fresh parsley
- 18 oz. peeled shrimp
- 1½ garlic cloves
- salt and pepper

Thousand island dip

- ¾ tbsp lemon juice
- 1½ tsp onion powder
- 1½ cups mayonnaise
- ¾ tbsp tomato paste
- 1½ tsp paprika powder
- 1½ tsp hot sauce
- salt and pepper

DIRECTIONS

In a bowl, place all the ingredients for the sauce and stir to combine.

Season with salt and pepper set aside.

In a skillet over medium-high heat, heat the oil or ghee. Crush the garlic cloves, but keep most of them in one piece. To flavor, the oil, add the crushed cloves but remove the cloves before serving.

Fry the shrimp in a skillet for 2-4 minutes on each side if using raw shrimp. As soon as they turn pink, they are ready. Toss in the chili flakes, salt, and pepper.

Shred the parsley and sprinkled over the top.

The fried shrimp are served immediately after being cooked along with the creamy dipping sauce.

NUTRITION:

Per Serving: Calories 98 | Protein 8g | Carbs 10g

SPINACH SAUCE

COOKING: 0 min   **PREPARATION:** 10 min   **SERVES:** 6

INGREDIENTS

- ¼ cup sour cream
- 2 tsp lemon juice
- 2 tbsp dried parsley
- ¼ tsp ground black pepper
- 1 tbsp dried dill
- 1 tsp onion powder
- 2 tbsp light olive oil
- ½ tsp salt
- 2 oz. frozen spinach
- 1 cup mayonnaise

DIRECTIONS

Let spinach thaw and be careful to remove excess liquid.

In a bowl, place the spinach and mix with all the other ingredients.

Upon obtaining a homogeneous mixture, let stand for 10-12 minutes to allow the flavors to develop

NUTRITION:

Per Serving: Calories 18 | Protein 5g | Carbs 2g

QUICK CRUNCHY TOAST

COOKING: 12 min **PREPARATION: 5 min** **SERVES: 8**

INGREDIENTS

- 1 cup almond flour
- 1 cup coconut flour
- 1/2 cup all-purpose flour
- 1/2 cup coconut oil, melted
- 1 cup sugar
- 1 teaspoon kosher salt
- 1 teaspoon cardamom
- 8 tablespoons coconut milk
- 1/4 teaspoon grated nutmeg
- 1 tablespoon cinnamon
- 3 tablespoons flaxseed, ground

DIRECTIONS

Preheat oven to 340 degrees F.
In a bowl, combine dry ingredients.
Add oil and milk and continue to mix.
Create a ball with the dough and roll it out between 2 sheets of baking paper.
Using a knife, cut into squares and prick them with a fork to prevent them from puffing up.
Bake in the preheated oven for about 12-15 minutes.
Serve.

NUTRITION:
Per Serving: Calories: 330 | Protein: 4g | Carbohydrates: 24g;

CHOCOLATE MOUSSE

COOKING: 0 min **PREPARATION: 5 min** **SERVES: 2**

INGREDIENTS

- 1/4 c. honey or your favorite keto sweetener
- 2 ripe avocados
- 1/2 c. chocolate chips melted
- 1 tsp. vanilla
- 3/4 c. heavy cream
- chocolate curls, for garnish
- 1/2 tsp. kosher salt
- 3 tbsp. unsweetened cocoa powder

DIRECTIONS

Place all ingredients in a blender, and blend until smooth.
When you are satisfied with the result transfer to serving glasses and let rest in the fridge for 40-50 minutes.
Garnish with chocolate curls as desired.

NUTRITION:
Per Serving: Calories 208 | Protein 4g | Carbs 36g

QUICK COOKIES SNACK

COOKING: 15 min   **PREPARATION: 5 min**   **SERVES: 15**

INGREDIENTS

- ¼ cup softened
- ⅓ cup granulated artificial sweetener
- 1 ¾ teaspoon water
- ☐ teaspoon salt
- ¼ cup semi-sweet chocolate chips
- ☐ teaspoon of vanilla extract
- ¼ cup chopped walnuts
- 1 egg, beaten
- 2 ☐ teaspoons whole-wheat flour
- ☐ teaspoon baking soda

DIRECTIONS

1. Preheat the oven to 350 degrees F.
2. In a bowl, cream together the butter and sweetener.
3. Stir in the egg, vanilla, and water.
4. Sift in the baking soda, salt, and flour and stir into the cream mixture.
5. Combine the walnuts and chocolate chips.
6. Drop the cookies by teaspoonfuls onto a baking sheet.
7. Bake in the oven for about 10-15 minutes.
8. Remove from baking sheet and allow to cool.

NUTRITION:
Per Serving: Calories 60 | Protein 4g | Carbohydrates 3g

CARAMEL PENUCHE

COOKING: 1 min   **PREPARATION: 5 min**   **SERVES: 12**

INGREDIENTS

- 4 ounces of dark vegan chocolate
- 1/2 cup almond milk
- 1 cup brown sugar
- 1/4 cup coconut oil, softened
- 1/2 cup walnuts, chopped
- 1/4 teaspoon cloves
- 1/2 teaspoon cinnamon powder

DIRECTIONS

Microwave chocolate until melted.
In a saucepan, heat the milk and add the hot milk to the melted chocolate.
Add remaining ingredients and stir to combine well, pour mixture into a well-greased baking dish and refrigerate until set.

NUTRITION:
Per Serving: Calories: 156 | Protein: 1g | Carbohydrates: 13g

TASTY CHOCOLATE CUSTARD

COOKING: 0 min | **PREPARATION: 10 min** | **SERVES: 2**

INGREDIENTS

- 1/4 cup of vegan half-and-half
- 2 tablespoons agave syrup
- 1/2 cup raw cashews, soaked and drained
- 4 tablespoons vegan chocolate chips
- 1/8 teaspoon coarse salt
- 1/8 teaspoon grated nutmeg
- 2 tablespoons coconut whipped cream

DIRECTIONS

Place cashews in the bowl of your high-speed blender. Add the remaining ingredients and blend until even and smooth. Pour mixture into 2 ramekins and refrigerate for at least 2 hours or until well chilled.
Garnish with coconut whipped cream and serve.

NUTRITION:
Per Serving: Calories: 288 | Protein: 10g | Carbohydrates: 47g

CHOCOLATE CHIA PUDDING

COOKING: 0 min | **PREPARATION: 10 min** | **SERVES: 4**

INGREDIENTS

- 4 tablespoons unsweetened cocoa powder
- 4 tablespoons of maple syrup
- 1 2/3 cups coconut milk
- A pinch of grated nutmeg
- A pinch of ground cloves
- 1/2 teaspoon ground cinnamon
- 1/2 cup chia seeds

DIRECTIONS

Add the maple syrup, milk the cocoa powder, and spices to a bowl, and mix until everything is well incorporated.
Add chia seeds and mix again to combine well. Pour the mixture into four jars, cover tightly, and refrigerate overnight. The next day, stir the mixture and enjoy!

NUTRITION:
Per Serving: Calories: 346 | Protein: 5g | Carbohydrates: 28g

FRESH AND QUICK VANILLA ICE CREAM

COOKING: 0 min   **PREPARATION: 10 min**   **SERVES: 4**

INGREDIENTS

- 1 cup coconut milk
- 1/4 cup agave syrup
- A pinch of ground aniseed
- 1/2 cup raw cashews, soaked overnight and drained
- A pinch of Himalayan salt
- 1 tablespoon of pure vanilla extract

DIRECTIONS

Place all ingredients in the bowl of your food processor or high-speed blender.
Blend ingredients until creamy, uniform, and smooth.
Place ice cream in the freezer for at least 3 hours.

NUTRITION:
Per Serving: Calories: 205 | Protein: 4g | Carbohydrates: 25g

APPLES AND ALMONDS PORRIDGE

COOKING: 15 min   **PREPARATION: 5 min**   **SERVES: 3**

INGREDIENTS

- 1 cup of toasted buckwheat
- 3/4 cup water
- 1 cup rice milk
- 1/4 teaspoon sea salt
- 3 tablespoons agave syrup
- 1 cup apples, diced and cored
- 3 tablespoons almonds, shelled
- 2 tablespoons coconut flakes
- 2 tablespoons hemp seeds

DIRECTIONS

In a saucepan, bring the water, milk, buckwheat semolina, and salt to a boil.
Lower the heat and stir until it thickens.
Stir in the agave syrup. Divide the oatmeal among three bowls.
Garnish each serving with apples, almonds, coconut, and hemp seeds.

NUTRITION:
Per Serving: Calories: 377 | Protein: 10g | Carbohydrates: 70g

VANILLA PROTEIN SHAKE

COOKING: 0 min | **PREPARATION: 5 min** | **SERVES: 2**

INGREDIENTS

- 2 tbsp almond butter
- 1 tsp ground cinnamon
- 1 cup coconut milk
- 2 tsp vanilla extract
- 2 oz. frozen cauliflower rice raw
- 8 tbsp pea unflavored protein powder
- 1 cup unsweetened almond milk

DIRECTIONS

Place ingredients in a blender.
Mix until smooth.
Pour into a tall glass and enjoy.

NUTRITION:

Per Serving: Calories 124 | Protein 22g | Carbs 25g

GREEK-STYLE FRUIT COMPOTE (HOSAFI)

COOKING: 15 min | **PREPARATION: 5 min** | **SERVES: 4**

INGREDIENTS

- 3 peaches, pitted and sliced
- 4 apricots, cut in half and pitted
- 4 dried apricots
- 1 cup dried figs
- 1 cup of sweet red wine
- 4 tablespoons of agave syrup
- 3-4 cloves
- 1 cinnamon stick
- 1 vanilla bean
- 1 cup whole coconut yogurt

DIRECTIONS

Add the fruit, dried fruit, wine, agave syrup, cloves, cinnamon, and vanilla in a saucepan and cover with 1-inch water. Bring to a boil and immediately reduce heat to a simmer.
Allow simmering, partially covered, for 15 minutes. Allow cooling completely.
Spoon into individual bowls and serve with well-chilled coconut yogurt.

NUTRITION:

Per Serving: Calories: 294 | Protein: 7g | Carbohydrates: 66g

STRAWBERRY SMOOTHIE

COOKING: 0 min   **PREPARATION: 3 min**   **SERVES: 4**

INGREDIENTS

- 10 oz. fresh strawberries sliced
- 1 tsp vanilla extract
- 2 tbsp lime juice
- 3½ cups unsweetened coconut milk

DIRECTIONS

In a blender, place all ingredients and blend until smooth. If you use coconut milk, you will get a creamier smoothie. Use more lime juice if desired.

NUTRITION:
Per Serving: Calories 108 | Protein 4g | Carbs 5g

HOMEMADE BREAKFAST CEREALS

COOKING: 15 min   **PREPARATION: 15 min**   **SERVES: 5**

INGREDIENTS

- 1 ½ cups of spelled flour
- 1/2 teaspoon baking powder
- 1 teaspoon cinnamon
- 1/2 teaspoon cardamom
- 1/4 teaspoon cloves
- 1/2 cup brown sugar
- 1/3 cup almond milk
- 2 teaspoons coconut oil, melted

DIRECTIONS

Preheating the oven to 350 degrees F.
In a bowl, thoroughly combine all dry ingredients.
Gradually, pour in the milk and coconut oil and stir to combine well.
Fill your pastry bag with the batter. Now, pipe 1/4-inch balls onto parchment cookie sheets.
Bake in the preheated oven for about 12-15 minutes. Serve with your favorite milk.
Store in a container with air for about 1 month.

NUTRITION:
Per Serving: Calories: 203 | Protein: 4g | Carbohydrates: 39g

CHEESECAKE WITH BLUEBERRIES

COOKING: 0 min **PREPARATION: 10 min** **SERVES: 12**

INGREDIENTS

- 1 cup almonds, ground
- 1 ½ cups dates, pitted
- 1 ½ cups vegan cream cheese
- 1/4 cup coconut oil, softened
- 1/2 cup fresh or frozen blueberries

DIRECTIONS

In your food processor, blend the almonds and 1 cup of dates until the mixture comes together; press the crust into a lightly greased muffin pan.

Then, blend the remaining 1/2 cup of dates together with the vegan cheese, coconut oil, and blueberries until creamy and smooth. Spoon the topping onto the crust.

Place these mini cheesecakes in the freezer for about 3 hours.

NUTRITION:

Per Serving: Calories: 235 | Protein: 4g | Carbohydrates: 17g;

SWEET SNACK PUDDING

COOKING: 10 min **PREPARATION: 5 min** **SERVES: 4**

INGREDIENTS

- 1 cup brown rice
- 1½ cups water - 1½ cups skimmed milk
- 3 tablespoons sugar (omit if using non-dairy sweetened milk)
- 2 teaspoons pumpkin spice or ground cinnamon
- 2 bananas
- 3 tablespoons chopped walnuts or sunflower seeds (optional)

DIRECTIONS

In a medium saucepan, combine the rice, water, milk, sugar, and pumpkin spice.

Bring to a boil over high heat, lower the heat to low, and cover the pot.

Simmer, occasionally stirring, until the rice is soft and the liquid has been absorbed.

Mash the bananas and mix them with the cooked rice. Serve topped with walnuts.

NUTRITION:

Per Serving: Calories 259 | Protein 8g | Carbohydrates 54g

SPICY COFFEE

COOKING: 3h | **PREPARATION: 10 min** | **SERVES: 7**

INGREDIENTS

- 4 cinnamon sticks, each about 3 inches long
- 1 1/2 teaspoons of whole cloves
- 1/3 cup of honey
- 2-ounce of chocolate syrup
- 1/2 teaspoon of anise extract
- 8 cups of brewed coffee

DIRECTIONS

Pour the coffee in a 4-quarts slow cooker, pour in the remaining ingredients except for cinnamon, and stir properly. Wrap the whole cloves in cheesecloth and tie its corners with strings.

Immerse this cheesecloth bag in the liquid present in the slow cooker and cover it with the lid.

Then plug in the slow cooker and let it cook on the low heat setting for 3 hours or until heated thoroughly. When done, discard the cheesecloth bag and serve.

NUTRITION:

Per Serving: Calories 150 | Protein 16g | Carbohydrates 21g

CARROT CAKE

COOKING: 10 min | **PREPARATION: 10 min** | **SERVES: 2**

INGREDIENTS

- ½ teaspoon, vanilla extract
- 1 cup water
- Salt
- 1 cup, non-dairy milk
- ¼ cup, raisins
- ½ cup, shredded carrots
- ¼ teaspoon, allspice
- ½ teaspoon, cinnamon
- 1 cup, rolled oats
- Toppings:
- 2 tablespoons, maple syrup
- ¼ cup, chopped walnuts
- 2 tablespoons, shredded coconut

DIRECTIONS

Place a small saucepan over low heat and bring non-dairy milk, oats, and water over low heat.

Now, add vanilla extract, carrots, cinnamon, raisins, salt, and allspice. Stir the mixture occasionally. You'll know they're ready when the liquid is fully absorbed into all the ingredients (in about 10 minutes).

Transfer the thickened dish to bowls. You can pour maple syrup on top or with coconut or nuts.

NUTRITION:

Per Serving: Calories 190 | Protein 3g | Carbohydrates 34g

THE PERFECT CEREAL BREAKFAST

COOKING: 0 min **PREPARATION: 10 min** **SERVES: 2**

INGREDIENTS

- ½ cup uncooked old-fashioned oatmeal
- ½ cup chopped dates
- 2 cups whole-grain cereal
- ¼ cup raisins
- ¼ cup almonds
- ¼ cup walnuts

DIRECTIONS

In a bowl, add all ingredients.
Store in an airtight container until ready to use.

NUTRITION:
Per Serving: Calories 60 | Protein 26g | Carbohydrates 12g

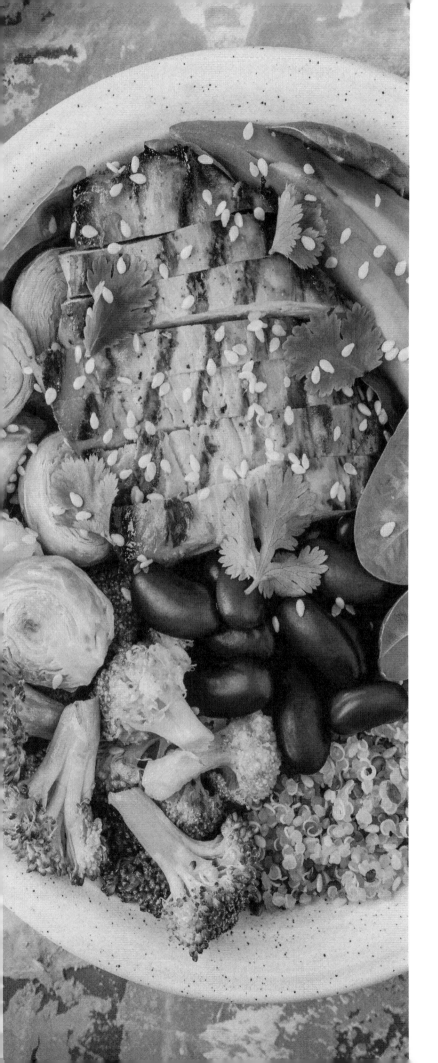

LUNCH RECIPES

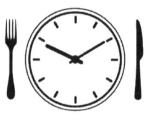

CLASSIC AVOCADO TOAST

COOKING: 15 min **PREPARATION: 10 min** **SERVES: 4**

INGREDIENTS

- 1 can, black beans
- Pinch, sea salt
- 2 pieces, whole-wheat toast
- ¼ teaspoon, chipotle spice
- Pinch, black pepper
- 1 teaspoon garlic powder
- 1 freshly juiced lime
- 1 freshly diced avocado
- ¼ cup, corn
- 3 tablespoons finely diced onion
- ½ freshly diced tomato
- Fresh cilantro

DIRECTIONS

Mix the chipotle spice with the beans, salt, garlic powder, and pepper. Add the lime juice.

In a saucepan, boil the mixture until smooth and thick.

In a bowl, mix the corn, tomato, avocado, red onion, cilantro, and juice from the rest of the lime.

Add a little pepper and salt.

Toast the bread and spread first the black bean mixture and then the avocado mixture.

NUTRITION:
Per Serving: Calories 290 | Protein 12g | Carbohydrates 34g

GREEK SALAD

COOKING: 0 min **PREPARATION: 10 min** **SERVES: 4**

INGREDIENTS

- ⅔ cucumber, sliced
- ⅔ cup crumbled feta cheese
- ⅔ green bell pepper, chopped
- ⅔ red bell pepper, chopped
- 1 ⅔ large tomatoes, chopped
- ¼ cup olive oil
- ☐ teaspoon dried oregano
- ⅔ lemon, squeezed
- Ground black pepper to taste
- ⅔ head of romaine lettuce - rinsed, dried, and chopped
- ⅔ red onion, thinly sliced
- ⅔ (6 ounces) can of pitted black olives

DIRECTIONS

Combine the tomatoes, onion, Romaine, peppers, cucumber, cheese, and olives in a large salad bowl.

Whisk together the oregano, olive oil, black pepper, and lemon juice. Pour the dressing over the salad, toss and serve.

NUTRITION:
Per Serving: Calories 255 | Protein 8g | Carbohydrates 34g

SAVORY MUFFINS

COOKING: 20 min **PREPARATION: 10 min** **SERVES: 2**

INGREDIENTS

- 2 whole-wheat English muffins separated
- ⅓ cup tomato salsa
- ¼ cup refried beans
- 1 small jalapeno, seeded and sliced
- ¼ cup onion, sliced
- 2 tablespoons diced plum or cherry tomato
- ⅓ cup vegan cheese shreds (pepper jack is delicious!)

DIRECTIONS

Preheat the oven to 380 F degrees and cover a baking sheet with aluminum foil.

Separate the English muffin and spread some of the sauce and beans.

Place some jalapenos and onions on top and sprinkle the cheese over everything.

Place on the baking sheet and bake for 20 minutes or until brown.

You can turn on the grill for a minute or two to melt the cheese.

NUTRITION:

Per Serving: Calories 196 | Protein 14g | Carbohydrates 23g

DELICIOUS SWEET SANDWICHES

COOKING: 0 min **PREPARATION: 5 min** **SERVES: 1**

INGREDIENTS

- ¼ cup, hot water
- 1 tablespoon, cinnamon
- ¼ cup, raisins
- 2 teaspoons, cacao powder
- 1 ripe banana
- 2 slices, whole-grain bread
- ¼ cup, natural peanut butter

DIRECTIONS

Mix cocoa powder, raisins, hot water, and cinnamon in a bowl.

Spread the peanut butter on the bread.

Cut up the bananas and place them on the toast.

Blend the raisin mixture and spread it on the sandwich in a blender.

NUTRITION:

Per Serving: Calories 85 | Protein 2g | Carbohydrates 14g

SIMPLE ITALIAN STYLE RISOTTO

COOKING: 20 min **PREPARATION: 10 min** **SERVES: 4**

INGREDIENTS

- ½ cup brown rice, rinsed
- 1 cup water
- ½ teaspoon dried basil
- 1 small onion, chopped
- 2 tablespoons raisins
- 5 ounces frozen peas, thawed
- ½ cup pecan halves, toasted
- 1 medium carrot, cut into matchsticks
- 4 green onions, cut into 1-inch pieces
- 1 tablespoon olive oil
- ½ teaspoon salt or to taste
- ½ teaspoon crushed red chili flakes or to taste
- Ground pepper or to taste

DIRECTIONS

Place a small saucepan with water over medium heat.
When it begins to boil, add the rice and basil. Stir.
Cook for 12 minutes until all the water is absorbed and the rice is cooked. Add more water if you think the rice is not cooked through.
Meanwhile, in a skillet over medium heat, place the raisins, onions, carrots, and sauté for about 5 minutes.
Add the pepper, peas, chili flakes, and salt.
Add the pecans and rice and stir.
Serve.

NUTRITION:
Per Serving: Calories 305 | Protein 8g | Carbohydrates 41g

VEGGIE RISOTTO

COOKING: 5 min **PREPARATION: 10 min** **SERVES: 8**

INGREDIENTS

- 2 tablespoons olive oil
- 4 cloves garlic, finely chopped
- 1.5 pounds Arborio rice
- 6 tomatoes, chopped
- 2 teaspoons chopped rosemary
- 6 courgettes, finely diced
- 1 ¼ cups peas, fresh or frozen
- 12 cups hot vegetable stock
- 1 cup chopped
- Salt to taste
- Freshly ground pepper

DIRECTIONS

Place a large skillet over medium heat. Add the oil and onion and sauté.
Add the tomatoes and cook until soft.
Add the rice and rosemary. Stir well.
Add half of the broth and cook until dry.
Add the remaining broth and cook for 5 minutes.
Add peas and zucchini and cook until rice is tender. Add salt and pepper to taste.
Stir in basil. Let stand for 10 minutes.

NUTRITION:
Per Serving: Calories 406 | Protein 14g | Carbohydrates 82g

THE SPINACH SOUP

COOKING: 25 min   **PREPARATION: 10 min**   **SERVES: 6**

INGREDIENTS

- 1 pound peeled and diced potatoes
- 1 tablespoon minced garlic
- 1 teaspoon dry mustard
- 6 cups vegetable broth
- 20 ounces chopped frozen spinach
- 2 cups chopped onion
- 1 ½ tablespoons salt
- ½ cup minced dill
- 1 cup basil
- ½ teaspoon ground black pepper

DIRECTIONS

Place and whisk the potatoes, mustard, onion, broth, garlic, and salt in a saucepan over medium-low heat.

When it starts to boil, lower the heat, cover with a lid, and cook for 25 minutes.

Add the remaining ingredients, blend and cook for a few more minutes, and serve.

NUTRITION:

Per Serving: Calories 165 | Protein 13g | Carbohydrates 12g

THE CURIOUS COCONUT SOUP

COOKING: 10 min   **PREPARATION: 15 min**   **SERVES: 4**

INGREDIENTS

- 1 teaspoon coconut oil
- 1 onion, diced
- ¾ cup coconut milk

DIRECTIONS

In a saucepan over medium heat, melt the coconut oil.

Add the onion and cook for about 5 minutes, then add the water and peas.

Bring to a boil, lower the heat and add the watercress, mint, salt, and pepper.

Cover and simmer for 5 minutes.

Add the coconut milk and blend the soup with an immersion blender.

NUTRITION:

Per Serving: Calories 178 | Protein 6g | Carbohydrates 18g

AUTUMN PUMPKIN SOUP

COOKING: 20 min **PREPARATION:** 20 min **SERVES:** 5

INGREDIENTS

- 2 cups pumpkin, diced
- 1/2 cup tomato, chopped
- 1/2 cup onion, chopped
- 1 1/2 tsp curry powder
- 1/2 tsp paprika
- 2 cups vegetable stock
- 1 tsp olive oil
- 1/2 tsp garlic, minced

DIRECTIONS

Add onion, garlic, and oil to a saucepan and sauté for about 5 minutes.
Add remaining ingredients to the saucepan and bring to a boil.
Reduce heat, cover, and simmer for 12 minutes.
Puree the soup with an immersion blender until smooth.
Serve warm.

NUTRITION:
Per Serving: Calories 70 | Protein 2g | Carbohydrates 14g

VEGETABLES SOUP

COOKING: 25 min **PREPARATION:** 10 min **SERVES:** 4

INGREDIENTS

- 1/2 cup unsweetened coconut milk
- 5 oz fresh spinach, chopped
- 5 watercress, chopped
- 8 cups vegetable stock
- 1 lb cauliflower, chopped

DIRECTIONS

In a saucepan over medium heat, add cauliflower and broth and bring to a boil for 10 minutes.
Add spinach and watercress and cook for another 15 minutes.
Remove from heat and blend the soup with an immersion blender.
Add the coconut milk and stir, then adjust the salt.
Stir well and serve hot.

NUTRITION:
Per Serving: Calories 153 | Protein 12g | Carbohydrates 9g

AVOCADO SOUP

COOKING: 0 min | **PREPARATION: 10 min** | **SERVES: 2**

INGREDIENTS

- 1 medium avocado, peeled, pitted, and cut into pieces
- 1 cup coconut milk
- 2 romaine lettuce leaves
- 20 fresh mint leaves
- 1 tbsp fresh lime juice
- 1/8 tsp salt

DIRECTIONS

In a blender, add all ingredients and blend until smooth. The soup should be thick.
Pour into serving bowls and refrigerate for 20 minutes.
Stir well and serve cold.

NUTRITION:

Per Serving: Calories 268 | Protein 3g | Carbohydrates 11g

BROCCOLI SALAD

COOKING: 0 min | **PREPARATION: 15 min** | **SERVES: 6**

INGREDIENTS

- 8 cups diced broccoli
- ¼ cup sunflower seeds
- 3 tablespoons apple cider vinegar
- ½ cup dried cranberries
- 1/3 cup cubed onion
- 1 cup mayonnaise
- ½ cup bacon bits
- 2 tablespoons sugar
- ½ teaspoon salt and ground black pepper

DIRECTIONS

Mix sugar, vinegar, pepper, mayonnaise, and salt in a bowl.
In another bowl, mix all remaining ingredients, pour in the prepared mayonnaise dressing, and mix well.
Chill in the refrigerator for 60 minutes.

NUTRITION:

Per Serving: Calories 276 | Protein 3g | Carbohydrates 22g

ORZO SALAD

COOKING: 20 min **PREPARATION: 5 min** **SERVES: 2**

INGREDIENTS

- 1 chopped onion
- 25g grated feta cheese
- 2 sliced bell peppers
- 1 tablespoon olive oil
- 6 sliced tomatoes
- 2 tablespoons chopped basil
- 25g orzo pasta

DIRECTIONS

Preheat the oven to a temperature of 350f.
Drizzle a baking sheet with olive oil, place peppers, onion, and drizzle again.
Bake for about 10 minutes.
Add the tomatoes and bake for another 8-10 minutes.
Meanwhile, cook the orzo according to the directions given on the package and cool it. Now toss them with the baked vegetables and drizzle with oil, cheese, basil, and serve.

NUTRITION:

Per Serving: Calories 422 | Protein 13g | Carbohydrates 52g

MODERN PASTA

COOKING: 10 min **PREPARATION: 15 min** **SERVES: 10**

INGREDIENTS

- 1-pound cooked pasta
- 2 diced broccoli florets
- 1 chopped onion
- 1 cup grated cheese
- 12 ounce cooked and finely chopped bacon
- ¾ teaspoon salt
- ¾ teaspoon ground black pepper
- 1 cup mayonnaise

DIRECTIONS

Mix all ingredients in a bowl and combine well.
Cover with plastic wrap and refrigerate for at least 1 hour.
Then serve.

NUTRITION:

Per Serving: Calories 461 | Protein 14g | Carbohydrates 36g

SANDWICHES

COOKING: 0 min **PREPARATION: 15 min** **SERVES: 4**

INGREDIENTS

- 1 pound extra-firm tofu drained and patted dry
- 1 medium red bell pepper, finely chopped
- 1 celery rib, finely chopped
- 3 green onions, minced
- ¼ cup shelled sunflower seeds
- ½ cup vegan mayonnaise, homemade or store-bought
- ½ teaspoon salt
- ½ teaspoon celery salt
- ¼ teaspoon freshly ground black pepper
- 8 slices whole-grain bread
- 4 (¼-inch) slices ripe tomato
- 4 lettuce leaves

DIRECTIONS

In a bowl, crumble the tofu.

Add sunflower seeds, bell pepper, onions, and celery. Add mayonnaise and mix until well combined.

Toast the bread, if desired. Spread mixture evenly over 4 slices of bread.

Top each with a tomato slice, a lettuce leaf, and the remaining bread. Cut the sandwiches in half diagonally and serve.

NUTRITION:

Per Serving: Calories 291 | Protein 16g | Carbohydrates 23g

BLACK BEAN

COOKING: 0 min **PREPARATION: 15 min** **SERVES: 8**

INGREDIENTS

- 2 15-ounce cans of black beans, rinsed and drained
- 1 jalapeno pepper, seeded and minced
- ½ of red bell pepper, seeded and diced
- ½ of yellow bell pepper, seeded and diced
- ½ of s small red onion, diced
- 1 cup fresh cilantro, finely chopped
- Zest of 1 lime
- Juice of 1 lime
- 1 10-ounce can Ro*tel, drained
- ½ teaspoon Kosher salt
- ¼ teaspoon ground black pepper

DIRECTIONS

Combine the garlic, cilantro, red and yellow bell pepper, green onions, beans, jalapeno, onion, and mix well.

Add the lime zest and juice, Ro-tel, salt, and pepper, and toss to combine.

Refrigerate for at least 2 hours before serving so that the flavors have time to blend. Serve with slices of wheat tortilla that have been crisped in the oven or with wheat or sesame crackers.

NUTRITION:

Per Serving: Calories 196 | Protein 12g | Carbohydrates 26g

SPECIAL CANNELLINI BEANS RECIPE

COOKING: 0 min **PREPARATION: 10 min** **SERVES: 8**

INGREDIENTS

- 1 15-ounce can cannellini beans, rinsed and drained
- ½ cup raw cashews
- 1 clove garlic, smashed
- 2 tablespoons diced, red bell pepper
- ½ teaspoon sea salt
- ¼ teaspoon cayenne pepper
- 4 teaspoons lemon juice
- 2 tablespoons water
- Dill sprigs or weed for garnish

DIRECTIONS

Combine the bell pepper, garlic, beans, and cashews in a bowl and pulse several times to break it up.

Add the water, salt, lemon juice, cayenne, and process until smooth.

Scrape into a bowl, cover, and refrigerate for at least 2 hours before serving. Garnish with fresh dill and serve with vegetable crackers.

NUTRITION:

Per Serving: Calories 203 | Protein 24g | Carbohydrates 36g

CUCUMBER LITTLE BITES

COOKING: 0 min **PREPARATION: 10 min** **SERVES: 2**

INGREDIENTS

- 1 cup raw sunflower seed
- ½ teaspoon salt
- ½ cup chopped fresh chives
- 1 clove garlic, chopped
- 2 tablespoons red onion, minced
- 2 tablespoons lemon juice
- ½ cup water (might need more or less)
- 4 large cucumbers

DIRECTIONS

Place the sunflower seeds and salt in the food processor and process until you have a fine powder. It will only take about 10 seconds.

Add the water, onion, chives, lemon juice, and garlic, and process until the mixture is smooth.

Cut the cucumbers into rounds.

Spread a tablespoon of the sunflower mixture over the top and place it on a serving dish.

Sprinkle with chopped chives and refrigerate until ready to serve.

NUTRITION:

Per Serving: Calories 203 | Protein 26g | Carbohydrates 41g

SPICY HUMMUS

COOKING: 0 min **PREPARATION: 10 min** **SERVES: 2**

INGREDIENTS

- 1 cup canned, unsweetened pumpkin puree
- 1 ounce can garbanzo beans, rinsed and drained
- 1 tablespoon apple cider vinegar
- 1 tablespoon maple syrup
- ¼ cup tahini
- 1 tablespoon fresh orange juice
- ½ teaspoon orange zest and additional zest for garnish
- ⅛ teaspoon ground cinnamon
- ⅛ teaspoon ground ginger
- ⅛ teaspoon ground nutmeg
- ¼ teaspoon salt

DIRECTIONS

Pour the pumpkin puree and garbanzo beans into a food processor and pulse to break up.
Add the vinegar, syrup, tahini, orange juice, and orange zest pulse a few times.
Add the cinnamon, ginger, nutmeg, and salt and process until smooth and creamy.
Serve in a bowl sprinkled with more orange zest with wheat crackers alongside.

NUTRITION:

Per Serving: Calories 154 | Protein 26g | Carbohydrates 14g

QUINOA MIX

COOKING: 10 min **PREPARATION: 10 min** **SERVES: 4**

INGREDIENTS

- 2 tablespoons ground flaxseed
- ⅓ cup unsweetened soy milk
- 1 cup old-fashioned rolled oats
- 1 cup cooked and cooled quinoa
- ¼ cup brown sugar
- 1 teaspoon ground cinnamon
- ¼ teaspoon salt
- ¼ cup pumpkin or sunflower seeds
- ¼ cup shredded coconut
- ½ cup almonds
- ½ cup raisins or dried cherries/cranberries

DIRECTIONS

Whisk the flax seeds and milk together in a small bowl and set aside for 20 minutes so the roots can absorb the milk.
Preheat the oven to 320 degrees F and coat a muffin pan with coconut oil.
Mix the oats, quinoa, brown sugar, cinnamon, salt, pumpkin seeds, coconut, almonds, and raisins in a large bowl.
Stir in flaxseed and milk mixture and combine thoroughly.
Place two generous teaspoons of the trail mix in each muffin cup. When done, wet your fingers and press down on each muffin cup to compact the trail mix.
Bake for 10 minutes.
Cool completely before removing, and each ramekin will fall.

NUTRITION:

Per Serving: Calories 185 | Protein 13g | Carbohydrates 32g

FRENCH OMELETTE

COOKING: 5 min   **PREPARATION: 5 min**   **SERVES: 2**

INGREDIENTS

- ¼ teaspoon, white pepper
- 1/3 cup, nutritional yeast
- ½ teaspoon, garlic powder
- ½ teaspoon, baking soda
- 3 green onions, finely chopped
- 4 ounces, sautéed mushrooms
- ½ teaspoon, onion powder
- ¼ teaspoon, black pepper
- 1 cup, chickpea flour

DIRECTIONS

Mix chickpea flour, white pepper, onion powder, garlic powder, black pepper, baking soda, and nutritional yeast in a small bowl.

Add 1 cup of water and create a smooth batter.

Heat a skillet and pour in the mixture.

On top of the batter, sprinkle some green onion and mushrooms. Flip the Omelette and cook evenly on both sides. Once both sides are cooked, serve the omelet with spinach, tomatoes, hot sauce, and salsa.

NUTRITION:

Per Serving: Calories 180 | Protein 10g | Carbohydrates 19g

CURRY CHICKPEAS

COOKING: 10 min   **PREPARATION: 5 min**   **SERVES: 6**

INGREDIENTS

- ¼ teaspoon of allspice
- 1 can of diced tomatoes
- 2 cans chickpeas, rinsed and drained
- Salt, cayenne pepper, to taste
- 1 tablespoon extra-virgin olive oil
- 1 yellow onion, diced
- 1 teaspoon curry

DIRECTIONS

In a skillet, simmer onions in 1 tablespoon oil for 5 minutes over medium heat.

Add the pepper and allspice and cook for 2 minutes.

Add the tomatoes and cook for another 2 minutes.

Add the chickpeas and simmer for 10 minutes.

Season with salt and serve.

NUTRITION:

Per Serving: Calories 168 | Protein 8g | Carbohydrates 33g

ITALIAN FARRO

COOKING: 40 min   **PREPARATION: 5 min**   **SERVES: 4**

INGREDIENTS

- ½ cup mushrooms, sliced
- 1½ teaspoons garlic powder
- 1½ teaspoons onion powder
- 1 cup zucchini, chopped
- 1 cup squash, chopped
- 1 red bell pepper, chopped
- ½ teaspoon paprika
- 4 cups potatoes, peeled and diced
- Salt and pepper, to taste
- 1 can of pinto beans, drained and rinsed
- Pinch of red pepper flakes

DIRECTIONS

Preheat oven to 400 degrees F.
Place the potatoes on a baking sheet and line it with baking paper.
Bake the potatoes for 20 minutes by placing the baking sheet in the oven.
Remove the baking sheet and add the zucchini, peppers, squash, beans, and mushrooms.
Sprinkle with the seasonings and bake for about 20 minutes.
Remove from oven and grab a large bowl.
Pour into the bowl and mix well.
Serve.

NUTRITION:
Per Serving: Calories 421 | Protein 5g | Carbohydrates 29g

THE PERFECT MUSHROOMS SIDE DISH

COOKING: 10 min   **PREPARATION: 5 min**   **SERVES: 4**

INGREDIENTS

- 1 tablespoon soy sauce
- 3 cloves garlic, minced
- ½ teaspoon thyme, chopped
- Salt and pepper, to taste
- 2 pounds mushrooms, sliced ¼ inch thick
- 2 tablespoons balsamic vinegar

DIRECTIONS

Mix soy sauce, balsamic vinegar, thyme, garlic, pepper, and salt in a bowl to make a marinade.
Allow mushrooms to marinate for 1 hour to 30 minutes.
Grill mushrooms over medium heat for 5 minutes on each side.
Serve and enjoy.

NUTRITION:
Per Serving: Calories 102; Protein 5g; Carbohydrates 19g

SPECIAL TOAST

COOKING: 2 min **PREPARATION: 5 min** **SERVES: 4**

INGREDIENTS

- 1 freshly squeezed lime
- 1 freshly diced avocado
- ¼ cup, corn
- ¼ teaspoon, chipotle spice
- Pinch, black pepper
- 1 teaspoon garlic powder
- 3 tablespoons finely chopped onion
- ½ fresh diced tomato
- Fresh cilantro
- 1 can, black beans
- Pinch, sea salt
- 2 pieces of whole-wheat toast

DIRECTIONS

Mix chipotle spice with salt, garlic powder, beans, and pepper. Add the lime juice.
Simmer until the mixture is thick and starchy.
Mix the red onion, tomato, corn, avocado, cilantro, and juice from the rest of the lime in a bowl. Season with pepper and salt.
Toast the bread and spread first the black bean mixture and then the avocado mix.
Serve.

NUTRITION:

Per Serving: Calories 285 | Protein 5g | Carbohydrates 26g

DELICIOUS SWEET BREAD

COOKING: 5 min **PREPARATION: 3 min** **SERVES: 2**

INGREDIENTS

- 2 teaspoons, cocoa powder
- 1 ripe banana
- 2 slices, whole wheat bread
- ¼ cup, natural peanut butter
- ¼ cup, hot water
- 1 tablespoon, cinnamon
- ¼ cup, raisins

DIRECTIONS

Mix the hot water, cinnamon, cocoa powder, and raisins in a bowl.
Spread the peanut butter on the bread.
Cut up the bananas and place them on the toast.
Mix the raisin mixture in a blender and spread it on the sandwich.

NUTRITION:

Per Serving: Calories 155 | Protein 2g | Carbohydrates 44g

MARINATED ANCHOVIES

COOKING: 10 min   **PREPARATION: 5 min**   **SERVES: 2**

INGREDIENTS

- 250g anchovies
- 5g olive oil
- 10g lemon juice
- 1 garlic
- parsley as you like

DIRECTIONS

Clean the anchovies; cut out some fillets and arrange them in a pan.

In a small bowl, emulsify the oil, lemon juice, garlic and parsley.

Pour the sauce over the dryers and leave to marinate for 20 minutes.

Cook in a pan until the anchovies are cooked and golden.

NUTRITION:

Per Serving: Calories 276 | Protein 23g | Carbohydrates 35g

TASTY RISOTTO

COOKING: 30 min   **PREPARATION: 15 min**   **SERVES: 6**

INGREDIENTS

- 6 zucchini, finely diced
- 1 ¼ cups peas, fresh or frozen
- 6 tomatoes, chopped
- 2 teaspoons rosemary, chopped
- 12 cups hot vegetable broth
- 1 cup chopped
- Salt to taste
- Freshly ground pepper
- 2 tablespoons olive oil
- 4 cloves garlic, finely chopped
- 1.5 pounds of Arborio rice

DIRECTIONS

Place a large heavy-bottomed skillet over medium heat. Add the oil. When oil is heated, add onion and sauté until translucent.

Add the tomatoes and cook until soft.

Add the rice and rosemary. Stir well.

Add half the broth and cook until liquid evaporates. Stir frequently.

Add the remaining broth and cook for 3-4 minutes.

Add peas and zucchini and cook until rice is tender. Season with salt and pepper to taste.

Stir in basil. Let stand for 5 minutes.

NUTRITION:

Per Serving: Calories 356 | Protein 2g | Carbohydrates 45g

DELICIOUS TOFU

COOKING: 35 min **PREPARATION: 5 min** **SERVES: 2**

INGREDIENTS

- 3 tablespoons dry barbecue rub
- ¼ cup barbecue sauce
- 1 block of hard or extra hard tofu
- 1 tablespoon mustard

DIRECTIONS

In a bowl, add dry BBQ rub, BBQ sauce, and mustard and mix.
Toss tofu in it to coat liberally.
Grill the tofu on a grill that is about 245 degrees F.
Cook for about 35 minutes.
Serve and enjoy.

NUTRITION:

Per Serving: Calories 108 | Protein 8g | Carbohydrates 12g

CRUNCHY ASPARAGUS

COOKING: 30 min **PREPARATION: 15 min** **SERVES: 5**

INGREDIENTS

- 1 bunch asparagus spears (about 12 spears)
- ¼ cup nutritional yeast
- 2 tablespoons hemp seeds
- 1 teaspoon garlic powder
- ¼ teaspoon paprika (or more if you like paprika)
- ⅛ teaspoon ground pepper
- ¼ cup whole-wheat breadcrumbs
- Juice of ½ lemon

DIRECTIONS

Preheat the oven to 330 degrees and line a baking sheet with baking paper.
Wash the asparagus, peeling off the white part at the bottom. Save them to make the vegetable broth.
Mix the paprika, bread crumbs, nutritional yeast, garlic powder, pepper, and hemp seeds together.
Arrange the asparagus spears on the baking sheets giving them some space, and sprinkle with the mixture in the bowl.
Bake for up to 30 minutes.
Serve with lemon juice, if desired.

NUTRITION:

Per Serving: Calories 196 | Protein 21g | Carbohydrates 34g

LIGHT BAKED FRIES

COOKING: 30 min **PREPARATION: 20 min** **SERVES: 4**

INGREDIENTS

- 1 pound potatoes, skins on, and cut into wedges
- 2 tablespoons sesame seeds
- 1 tablespoon potato starch
- 1 tablespoon sesame oil
- Salt to taste
- Black pepper to taste

DIRECTIONS

Preheat the oven to 370 degrees F and cover a baking sheet with baking paper.

Cut up the potatoes and place them in a large bowl.

Add the potato starch, sesame seeds, pepper, sesame oil, and salt.

Mix with your hands and make sure all the wedges are coated.

Spread the potato wedges on the baking sheets with a bit of space between each clove.

Bake for 20 minutes, turn the wedges over and return them to the oven for another 10 minutes until they appear golden brown.

NUTRITION:

Per Serving: Calories 210; Protein 21g; Carbohydrates 13g

YUMMY KALE CHIPS

COOKING: 30 min **PREPARATION: 5 min** **SERVES: 4**

INGREDIENTS

- 4 cloves garlic
- 1 cup olive oil
- 8 to 10 cups fresh kale, chopped
- 1 tablespoon of garlic-flavored olive oil
- ½ teaspoon garlic salt
- ½ teaspoon pepper
- 1 pinch red pepper flakes (optional)

DIRECTIONS

Peel and crush the garlic clove and place it in a small jar with a lid.

Pour the olive oil on top, cover tightly, and shake.

Drain the garlic and save the oil when you're ready to use it.

Preheat the oven to 200 degrees F.

Place the kale on a baking sheet, sprinkle with red pepper flakes, pepper, and garlic salt, then drizzle with olive oil.

Bake for 30 minutes, remove from oven and let chips cool.

NUTRITION:

Per Serving: Calories 310 | Protein 30g | Carbohydrates 24g

SQUASH SOUP

COOKING: 20 min | **PREPARATION: 10 min** | **SERVES: 6**

INGREDIENTS

- 4 cups water
- 1 garlic clove
- 1 tablespoon dried onion flakes
- 1 tablespoon curry powder
- 1 teaspoon kosher salt
- 3 cups butternut squash, chopped
- 1 ½ cups unsweetened coconut milk
- 1 tablespoon coconut oil

DIRECTIONS

Add the coconut oil, butternut squash, curry powder, water, onion flakes, garlic, and salt to a large saucepan,
Bring to a boil over high heat.
Lower the heat to medium and simmer for 15 minutes.
Puree the soup with an immersion blender until smooth and homogeneous. Return the soup to the pot, stir in the coconut milk and cook for 2 minutes.
Stir well and serve hot.

NUTRITION:
Per Serving: Calories 125; Protein 2g; Carbohydrates 14g

MILLET AND MIX

COOKING: 20 min | **PREPARATION: 5 min** | **SERVES: 2**

INGREDIENTS

- 1 cup millet
- ½ cup teff wheat
- 4 ½ cups water
- 1 onion, sliced
- 1 butternut squash, chopped
- Sea salt, to taste

DIRECTIONS

Rinse the millet and place it in a large pot.
Add the wheat, onion, pumpkin, salt, and water. Stir well.
Simmer for 20 minutes until all the water is absorbed.
Serve hot.

NUTRITION:
Per Serving: Calories 213 | Protein 9g | Carbohydrates 7g

SUMMER PIZZA

COOKING: 15 min **PREPARATION: 10 min** **SERVES: 2**

INGREDIENTS

- ½ cup corn kernels, cooked
- ½ cup beans, cooked
- ½ cup fire-roasted red peppers, chopped
- 1 Lavash flatbread, whole wheat
- 4 tablespoons cream of feta cheese, store-bought
- ½ cup cheddar cheese, shredded

DIRECTIONS

Preheat oven to 340ºF.
Cut Lavash into two halves. Bake crusts on a baking sheet in the oven for 5 minutes. Spread feta cheese on both crusts. Top with cheddar, corn kernels, red peppers, and beans. Bake for an additional 10 minutes.

NUTRITION:

Per Serving: Calories 558 | Protein 2g | Carbohydrates 64g

HOT WRAP

COOKING: 25 min **PREPARATION: 10 min** **SERVES: 4**

INGREDIENTS

- 1 avocado, diced
- 1 cup new potatoes, thinly sliced - ½ cup salsa
- 1 cup roasted green chilli, cut into strips
- 4 burrito wraps
- 1 cup black beans, washed and drained
- Sea salt and black pepper, as needed
- Fresh cilantro leaves, chopped
- 12 ounces of extra firm tofu - 1 teaspoon of cumin, ground
- 1 garlic clove, minced

DIRECTIONS

First heat the oil in a large pot over medium-high heat. Once the oil gets hot, stir in the potatoes and roasted green chilli strips.
Cook until cooked through and golden brown. Transfer the potato mixture to a plate and then add the tofu to the pan. Next, mash the tofu with a potato masher and cook for 4 to 5 minutes or until golden brown.
Put the potato and green chilli mixture back into the pan and give everything a good stir. After that, add the cumin, salt, pepper and garlic. Cook for a further 5 minutes.
Finally, heat up the sauce and the burrito wraps. Spread the sauce over the wraps. Add the tofu the potato mixture, the avocado and the cilantro, and wrap your burrito.
Serve hot and enjoy.

NUTRITION:

Per Serving: Calories 311 | Protein 20g | Carbohydrates 31g

HEALTHY TURKEY PASTA

COOKING: 10 min   **PREPARATION: 10 min**   **SERVES: 6**

INGREDIENTS

- ¾ package of spring lettuce
- 2½ teaspoons grape tomatoes halved
- 2 teaspoons minced fresh garlic
- ⅓ cup red wine vinegar
- 2 ¾ teaspoons olive oil
- 1 ½ teaspoons dried oregano
- ¼ cup Turkey Breast
- ¼ cup cooked penne pasta
- ⅓ cup thinly sliced red onions
- 6 ounces of crumbled feta cheese
- ¾ tin of pitted, drained, chopped olives
- ⅓ cup chopped Italian parsley

DIRECTIONS

1. In a bowl, combine oregano, olive oil, garlic, vinegar, and mix well, then set aside.
2. In a bowl combine the remaining ingredients.
3. Gently stir in dressing.
4. Serve.

NUTRITION:
Per Serving: Calories 350 | Protein 21g | Carbohydrates 24g

PESTO PITA

COOKING: 10 min   **PREPARATION: 10 min**   **SERVES: 4**

INGREDIENTS

- 4 small tomatoes, chopped
- 4 Greek pita flatbreads
- 16 pitted olives
- ¼ cup of prepared pesto
- 1 cup feta cheese

DIRECTIONS

Preheat oven to 290 degrees F.
Take the pita bread and spread the pesto on each one.
Also, add the olives, tomatoes, and feta cheese.
Place each pita on a tray to place in the oven.
Bake for about 10 minutes. The cheese should be melted.

NUTRITION:
Per Serving: Calories 440 | Protein 18g | Carbohydrates 37g

BRUSSELS AND BLUEBERRY SALAD

COOKING: 0 min **PREPARATION: 10 min** **SERVES: 6**

INGREDIENTS

- 3 tablespoons lemon juice
- ¼ cup olive oil
- Salt and pepper to taste
- 1 pound Brussels sprouts, thinly sliced
- ¼ cup dried blueberries, chopped
- ½ cup pecans, toasted and chopped
- ½ cup Parmesan cheese, cut into rounds

DIRECTIONS

Mix olive oil, lemon juice, salt, and pepper in a bowl.
Dip the Brussels sprouts, blueberries, and pecan into this mixture.
Sprinkle the parmesan cheese on top.

NUTRITION:
Per Serving: Calories 245 | Protein 6g | Carbohydrates 15g

POTATO LATKE

COOKING: 10 min **PREPARATION: 15 min** **SERVES: 6**

INGREDIENTS

- 3 eggs, beaten
- 1 onion, grated
- 1 ½ teaspoons baking powder
- Salt and pepper to taste
- 2 pounds potatoes, peeled and grated
- ¼ cup all-purpose flour
- 4 tablespoons vegetable oil
- Chopped chives

DIRECTIONS

Preheat oven to 400 degrees F.
Beat eggs, baking powder, onion, salt, and pepper in a bowl.
Wipe the moisture from the shredded potatoes using a paper towel.
Add the potatoes to the egg mixture. Stir in flour.
Pour the oil into a frying pan over medium heat.
Cook a small amount of batter for 3 to 4 minutes per side.
Repeat until the rest of the battery runs out.
Garnish with chives.

NUTRITION:
Per Serving: Calories 216 | Protein 6g | Carbohydrates 29g

QUICK BROCCOLI RABE

COOKING: 15 min | **PREPARATION: 15 min** | **SERVES: 6**

INGREDIENTS

- 2 oranges, cut in half
- 1 pound broccoli rabe
- 2 tablespoons sesame oil, toasted
- Salt and pepper to taste
- 1 tablespoon sesame seeds, toasted

DIRECTIONS

Pour the oil into a frying pan over medium heat.
Add the oranges and cook until caramelized.
Transfer to a plate.
Place the broccoli in the pan and cook for 10 minutes.
Squeeze the oranges to obtain the juice in a bowl.
Mix in the salt, oil, and pepper.
Coat the broccoli rabe with the mixture.
Sprinkle with seeds.

NUTRITION:
Per Serving: Calories 59 | Protein 2g | Carbohydrates 4g

EVERYGREEN PUMPKIN SEED GRANOLA

COOKING: 30 min | **PREPARATION: 10 min** | **SERVES: 2**

INGREDIENTS

- ¼ cup chia seeds
- ¼ cup coconut oil, melted
- 3 cups rolled oats
- A pinch of salt
- ½ cup whole wheat flour - ½ teaspoon cinnamon
- ½ cup maple syrup - 2/3 cup pumpkin seeds
- ¼ cup coconut palm sugar
- ½ cup dry, unsweetened coconut flakes
- 1 cup broken red lentils, cooked
- 2/3 cup buckwheat groats

DIRECTIONS

Preheat oven to 375°F. Then, stir together the oats, cinnamon, flour, coconut sugar, pumpkin seeds, buckwheat groats, chia seeds, and coconut in a bowl.
Then, add the maple syrup, melted coconut oil, coconut sugar, and red lentils. Stir until everything is well combined.
Then, transfer the nut and cereal mixture to a greased and lined baking tray and spread it out evenly. Bake the mixture for 10 minutes.
Take out the baking tray and stir in the granola, then bake for 10 minutes and repeat this process. Finally, bake for 15 minutes.
Cool the granola completely before storing it in an airtight container.

NUTRITION:
Per Serving: Calories 362 | Protein 11g | Carbohydrates 48g

DELICIOUS WHIPPED POTATOES

COOKING: 35 min   **PREPARATION:** 10 min   **SERVES:** 6

INGREDIENTS

- 4 cups water
- 3 lb. potatoes, diced
- 3 cloves of garlic, crushed 6 tbsp. butter
- 2 bay leaves 10 sage leaves
- ½ cup Greek yogurt ¼ cup low-fat milk
- Salt to taste

DIRECTIONS

Boil the potatoes in water for 30 minutes. Drain. Use a fork to mash the potatoes.

In a frying pan over medium heat, cook garlic in butter for 1 minute. Add the sage and cook for a further 5 minutes. Discard the garlic.

Add the mashed potatoes, butter, yogurt, and milk to a bowl. Mix everything together and whisk with an electric mixer. Season with salt.

NUTRITION:
Per Serving: Calories 169 | Protein 4g | Carbohydrates 22g

AVOCADO QUINOA SALAD

COOKING: 4 min   **PREPARATION:** 15 min   **SERVES:** 4

INGREDIENTS

- 2 tablespoons balsamic vinegar
- ¼ cup of cream
- ¼ cup buttermilk
- 5 tablespoons freshly squeezed lemon juice, separated
- 1 clove of garlic, grated
- 2 tablespoons chopped shallots
- Salt and pepper to taste
- 2 tablespoons avocado oil, divided
- 1 ¼ cups quinoa, cooked
- 2 heads of endive, sliced
- 2 hard-boiled pears, thinly sliced
- 2 avocados, sliced
- ¼ cup fresh dill, chopped

DIRECTIONS

Combine cream, vinegar, milk, garlic, shallots, 1 tablespoon lemon juice, salt, and pepper in a bowl.

Pour 1 tablespoon oil into a frying pan over medium heat. Heat the quinoa for 5 minutes and transfer to a plate.

Stir the endive and pears into the mixture of lemon juice, remaining oil, salt, and pepper.

Transfer to a plate.

Toss the avocado in the reserved dressing. Add to the dish. Cover with the dill and quinoa.

NUTRITION:
Per Serving: Calories 431 | Protein 6 | Carbohydrates 22g

QUICK CAULIFLOWER SALAD

COOKING: 15 min **PREPARATION: 10 min** **SERVES: 4**

INGREDIENTS

- 8 cups of cauliflower florets
- 5 tablespoons olive oil, divided
- Salt and pepper to taste
- 1 cup parsley
- 1 clove of garlic, minced
- 2 tablespoons lemon juice
- ¼ cup almonds, toasted and sliced
- 3 cups arugula
- 2 tablespoons olives, sliced
- ¼ cup feta, crumbled

DIRECTIONS

Preheat oven to 430 degrees F.
Season the cauliflower in a mixture of 1 tablespoon olive oil, salt and pepper.
Place in a baking dish and roast for 15 minutes.
Put the remaining oil, lemon juice, parsley, garlic, salt, and pepper in a blender.
Pulse until smooth.
Put the roasted cauliflower in a salad bowl, and mix the rest of the ingredients with the parsley dressing.

NUTRITION:
Per Serving: Calories 198 | Protein 5g | Carbohydrates 10g

DELICIOUS POTATOES AND TURNIPS

COOKING: 30 min **PREPARATION: 5 min** **SERVES: 6**

INGREDIENTS

- 1 head of garlic
- 1 teaspoon of olive oil
- 1 pound turnips, diced
- 2 lbs potatoes, diced
- ½ cup almond milk
- ½ cup Parmesan cheese, grated
- 1 tablespoon fresh thyme, chopped
- 1 tablespoon fresh chives, chopped
- 2 tablespoons butter
- Salt and pepper to taste

DIRECTIONS

Boil the turnips and potatoes in a pot of water for 30 minutes.
Meanwhile, add the garlic, oil, milk, thyme, chives, salt, and pepper to a food processor.
Pulse until smooth.
Plate the turnips together with the puree and enjoy.

NUTRITION:
Per Serving: Calories 141 | Protein 4g | Carbohydrates 24g

COD STEW WITH RICE

COOKING: 30 min **PREPARATION: 10 min** **SERVES: 4**

INGREDIENTS

- 2 cups water
- ¾ cup brown rice 1 tablespoon vegetable oil
- 1 tablespoon ginger, chopped
- 1 tablespoon chopped garlic
- 1 sweet potato, diced
- 1 pepper, sliced 1 tablespoon curry powder
- Salt to taste
- 15 ounces of coconut milk 4 cod fillets
- 2 teaspoons freshly squeezed lime juice
- 3 tablespoons cilantro, chopped

DIRECTIONS

Put the water and rice in a saucepan, bring to a boil and then simmer for 15 minutes. Set aside.

Pour the oil into a frying pan over medium heat, add the garlic and cook for 30 seconds. Add the sweet potatoes and pepper. Season with curry powder and salt. Pour in the coconut milk and simmer for 10 minutes.

Add the fish to the sauce and cook for a further 8 minutes. Stir in the lime juice and coriander.

Serve with rice.

NUTRITION:

Per Serving: Calories 382 | Protein 19g | Carbohydrates 35g

RAW ZOODLES

COOKING: 0 min **PREPARATION: 10 min** **SERVES: 2**

INGREDIENTS

- 1 medium courgette
- 1½ cups basil
- 1/3 cup water
- 5 tablespoons pine nuts
- 2 tablespoons lemon juice
- 1 medium avocado, peeled, pitted, sliced
- 2 tablespoons olive oil
- 6 yellow cherry tomatoes, halved
- 6 red cherry tomatoes, halved
- Sea salt and black pepper to taste

DIRECTIONS

Add the lemon juice, olive oil, water, walnuts, basil, avocado slices, salt, and pepper to a blender.

Blend ingredients until smooth.

Add the halved yellow tomatoes and red tomatoes to the mixture; divide the sauce and sliced courgettes between two medium-sized serving bowls, and combine in each.

Serve and enjoy!

NUTRITION:

Per Serving: Calories 317 | Protein 7g | Carbohydrates 6g

SANDWICH WITH ARTICHOKE AND WHITE BEANS

COOKING: 0 min   **PREPARATION: 10 min**   **SERVES: 2**

INGREDIENTS

- ½ cup raw cashews, chopped
- Water
- 1 garlic clove, cut in half
- 1 tablespoon lemon zest
- 1 teaspoon fresh rosemary, chopped
- ¼ teaspoon salt
- ¼ teaspoon pepper
- 6 tablespoons almond, soya, or coconut milk
- 1 15.5-ounce can of cannellini beans, rinsed and well-drained
- 3 or 4 canned artichoke hearts, chopped
- ¼ cup hulled sunflower seeds
- Green onions, chopped, for garnish

DIRECTIONS

Soak raw cashews for 15 minutes in water. Drain and pat dry with a paper towel.

Transfer the cashews to a blender and add the garlic, lemon zest, rosemary, salt, and pepper. Pulse to break everything down and add the milk until the mixture is smooth and creamy.

Mash the beans in a bowl with a fork. Add the artichoke hearts and sunflower seeds. Stir to combine.

Pour the cashew mixture over the top. Mix ingredients well and spread on wholemeal bread.

NUTRITION:

Per Serving: Calories 110 | Protein 6g | Carbohydrates 14g

PINWHEELS OF FETA CHEESE AND SPINACH

COOKING: 30 min   **PREPARATION: 5 min**   **SERVES: 4**

INGREDIENTS

- 1 medium onion, finely chopped
- 3 tablespoons olive oil
- 2 tablespoons dried oregano
- 1 garlic clove, minced
- 3 packages frozen chopped spinach, thawed and squeezed
- 3 cups crumbled feta cheese
- 3 eggs, lightly beaten
- 1 package of puff pastry

DIRECTIONS

Place the oil in a skillet over medium-high heat and sauté the onion.

Add the oregano and garlic and cook for 2 minutes, then add the spinach cook for about five more minutes. Transfer to a bowl and let cool.

Add the spinach, eggs, and feta cheese to the spinach;

Open the puff pastry and spread each sheet with half of the spinach mixture to the edges.

Roll up the puff pastry and cut it into slices.

Bake in the oven at 350° for about 30 minutes. Serve warm.

NUTRITION:

Per Serving: Calories 205 | Protein 8g | Carbohydrates 17g

GREEN OLIVES TOASTED BREAD

COOKING: 0 min **PREPARATION: 5 min** **SERVES: 16**

INGREDIENTS

- 3 cups of olives
- 2 teaspoons of lemon juice
- 16 slices of toasted French bread
- 1 cup olive oil
- 1 garlic clove, peeled
- 1/4 teaspoon pepper
- 3 anchovy fillets
- A pinch of sugar
- 1/4 teaspoon salt

DIRECTIONS

Place all ingredients except the olives and bread in a food processor and combine. Process until smooth.
Add the chopped olives.
Serve with toasted French bread.

NUTRITION:

Per Serving: Calories 120 | Protein 2g | Carbohydrates 9g

PROTEIN CHICKEN WITH RICE AND TOMATO

COOKING: 15 min **PREPARATION: 20 min** **SERVES: 6**

INGREDIENTS

- 1 cup of water
- 4 tablespoons of tomato paste
- 1 tablespoon lemon juice
- 1 teaspoon salt
- 2 teaspoon chili powder
- 1/2 teaspoon garlic powder
- 1/2 teaspoon ginger powder
- 1 teaspoon ground
- Chopped fresh parsley
- fennel seeds
- 1/4 teaspoon turmeric powder
- 1 teaspoon ground coriander, optional
- 4 tablespoons olive oil
- 1 onion, chopped
- 2 pounds boneless, skinless chicken breasts
- 4 cups hot cooked rice

DIRECTIONS

In a bowl, mix the tomato paste, water, lemon juice, chili powder, salt, garlic powder, turmeric, fennel, cilantro, and ginger until smooth.
Heat the oil in a skillet over medium-high heat and add the onions;
Add the chicken as well and cook for about 5 minutes.
Pour the water mixture into a skillet.
Simmer uncovered for about 10 minutes.
Serve with rice. If desired, add parsley.

NUTRITION:

Per Serving: Calories 203 | Protein 12g | Carbohydrates 43g

COUSCOUS WITH OLIVES AND BEANS

COOKING: 15 min **PREPARATION: 10 min** **SERVES: 6**

INGREDIENTS

- 15 ounces chopped artichoke hearts
- 2 cloves of garlic, minced
- 1 can of chickpeas or beans, rinsed and drained
- 1 cup whole couscous
- 2 tablespoon olive oil
- A pinch of pepper
- 2 cups water
- 1 tablespoon lemon juice
- 1 medium onion, chopped
- A bit of cayenne pepper
- 1 can stewed tomatoes, chopped
- 1 cup pitted Greek olives, chopped
- 1/2 teaspoon dried oregano

DIRECTIONS

Bring water to a boil in a saucepan. Stir in the couscous. When cooked, remove from heat and let stand for about 10 minutes.
Meanwhile, heat oil over medium-high heat in a nonstick skillet.
When hot, add the onion and sauté.
Then add the garlic and cook for 2 more minutes.
Add the remaining ingredients, stirring a few times.
Serve with couscous.

NUTRITION:

Per Serving: Calories 340 | Protein 11g | Carbohydrates 51g

OMELET WITH BROCCOLI

COOKING: 15 min **PREPARATION: 10 min** **SERVES: 5**

INGREDIENTS

- 3 cups fresh broccoli florets
- 7 large eggs
- 1/2 cup milk
- 1/2 teaspoon salt
- 1/2 teaspoon pepper
- 1/2 cup grated Romano cheese
- 1/2 cup sliced pitted olives
- 2 tablespoons olive oil
- A little fresh chopped parsley

DIRECTIONS

Place the steamer basket in a casserole dish. Place the broccoli in the basket. Bring the water to a boil and steam for about 5 minutes.
In a bowl, place milk and whisk in eggs, salt and pepper. Add to cooked broccoli, grated cheese, and olives.
Heat oil in a skillet over medium heat and pour in egg mixture. Cook without lid for about 4 minutes or until eggs are set.
Let stand 5 minutes, cut into wedges and sprinkle with parsley and cheese.

NUTRITION:

Per Serving: Calories 217; Protein 16g; Carbohydrates 7g

ROASTED VEGETABLES

COOKING: 35 min | **PREPARATION: 5 min** | **SERVES: 5-6**

INGREDIENTS

- 10 garlic cloves, peeled
- 12 ounces potatoes cut in half or cubed
- 12 ounces of tomatoes
- 1 tablespoon dried oregano
- 8 ounces of mushrooms
- 2 zucchini cut
- 1/2 teaspoon salt
- 1/2 teaspoon pepper
- Extra virgin olive oil
- Fresh grated Parmesan cheese
- 1 teaspoon dried thyme

DIRECTIONS

Preheat oven to 370 degrees F.
In a bowl, place the vegetables, mushrooms, and garlic. Drizzle with olive oil, then add while stirring the thyme, dried oregano, pepper, and salt.
Spread the potatoes on a baking sheet and drizzle with oil.
Bake in the heated oven for 15 minutes. Remove from oven and add vegetables and mushrooms.
Return to the oven for another 20 minutes.
Sprinkle with grated Parmesan cheese and serve.

NUTRITION:

Per Serving: Calories 110 | Protein 23g | Carbohydrates 13g

ROASTED TOMATOES WITH PARMESAN

COOKING: 25 min | **PREPARATION: 10 min** | **SERVES: 4**

INGREDIENTS

- 4 tomatoes, halved
- 2 tablespoon olive oil
- 1 pinch of salt
- Ground black pepper to taste
- 1 cup grated Parmesan cheese

DIRECTIONS

Preheat oven to 340 degrees F.
Place tomatoes in a bowl and season with salt, pepper and olive oil.
Arrange the tomatoes on a baking sheet and sprinkle with the parmesan cheese.
Bake in the preheated oven for about 25 minutes.
Let cool for 5 minutes and serve.

NUTRITION:

Per Serving: Calories 67; Protein 5g; Carbohydrates 4g

ROASTED PEPPERS

COOKING: 25 min   **PREPARATION: 15 min**   **SERVES: 10-12**

INGREDIENTS

- 2 green peppers, cut in half
- 2 red peppers, cut in half
- olive oil cooking spray
- 2 teaspoons salt
- 2 yellow peppers, cut in half
- 1 teaspoon freshly ground black pepper
- ¼ cup cherry tomatoes halved
- 1 cup fresh basil, chopped
- 2 tablespoons herb vinegar
- 16 garlic cloves, thinly sliced

DIRECTIONS

Preheat the oven to 380 degrees F and grease a baking sheet with olive oil cooking spray.
Place the bell pepper halves on the baking sheet with the open side up.
Mix the garlic, basil, and cherry tomatoes in a bowl.
Then place the created mix into each bell pepper half and season with salt and pepper.
Cover the baking dish with aluminum foil and place it in the preheated oven.
Bake for 10 minutes, remove the aluminum foil and bake for about 15 minutes.
Remove from oven and drizzle with herb vinegar.

NUTRITION:
Per Serving: Calories 19; Protein 1g; Carbohydrates 4g

GREEN SOUP

COOKING: 20 min   **PREPARATION: 10 min**   **SERVES: 6**

INGREDIENTS

- 3 yellow squash, diced
- 1 ½ tomato, diced
- 3 zucchini, diced
- 1 ½ pinch of garlic and pepper
- ⅓ cup and 2 teaspoons fresh mushrooms, sliced
- 2 tablespoons olive oil

DIRECTIONS

In a skillet over medium heat, place 2 tablespoons of olive oil, the garlic, and then add the tomatoes.
Cook for 5 minutes and add pepper.
Add the squash, zucchini, and mushrooms.
Lower the heat and cook for about 10-15 minutes

NUTRITION:
Per Serving: Calories 66 | Protein 4g | Carbohydrates 13g

CORN PEPPERS SALAD

COOKING: 10 min | **PREPARATION: 10 min** | **SERVES: 3**

INGREDIENTS

- ¼ bunch of fresh cilantro, chopped, or more to taste
- 1 teaspoon olive oil
- ½ green bell pepper, diced
- 1 large tomato, diced
- salt and ground black pepper to taste
- 3 ears of freshly shelled corn
- 2 tablespoons red onion, diced

DIRECTIONS

Grease a grill with oil and preheat to medium heat.
Place the corn on the grill and cook for about 10 minutes, taking care to turn them occasionally while cooking.
After they are cooked, in a bowl, combine and mix the hot corn kernels with the green bell pepper, oil, onion, diced tomato, cilantro, salt, and pepper.
Set aside for 1 hour for flavors to meld.
Serve.

NUTRITION:

Per Serving: Calories 103 | Protein 4g | Carbohydrates 20g

LIGHT ASPARAGUS

COOKING: 8 min | **PREPARATION: 10 min** | **SERVES: 6**

INGREDIENTS

- 1 pinch of salt and pepper to taste
- 1 ½ tablespoon extra-virgin olive oil
- 1 tablespoon chopped garlic
- 1 ½ pound thin asparagus, trimmed and cut in half
- 1 ½ large tomato, chopped

DIRECTIONS

In a skillet over high heat, place the water and asparagus.
Cover the pan. When the water comes to a boil, cook until the asparagus is tender.
In another skillet over medium heat, put the oil and garlic.
Cook and stir for about 2 minutes.
Add the tomato, salt, and pepper and cook for about 2 minutes.
Also, add the asparagus to the skillet and cook for another 2 minutes.
Serve hot.

NUTRITION:

Per Serving: Calories 63 | Protein 4g | Carbohydrates 7g

TUNA SALAD

COOKING: 0 min | **PREPARATION: 5 min** | **SERVES: 8**

INGREDIENTS

- ½ cup finely chopped red onion
- 5 ounces drained light tuna pieces
- ½ teaspoon ground black pepper
- ½ cup chopped fresh parsley
- 1 teaspoon lemon zest
- ½ teaspoon salt
- 3 teaspoons olive oil
- ¼ cup freshly squeezed lemon juice

DIRECTIONS

In a bowl, put together the parsley, onion, and tuna.
After mixing, put in the salt, lemon juice, oil, lemon zest, and pepper.
Mix well and serve.

NUTRITION:
Per Serving: Calories 169 | Protein 17g | Carbohydrates 3g

BAKED MEDITERRANEAN SALMON

COOKING: 15 min | **PREPARATION: 20 min** | **SERVES: 6**

INGREDIENTS

- 1 cup balsamic vinegar
- 6 cloves garlic, crushed
- 3 teaspoons fresh basil, chopped
- ¾ cup olive oil
- 6 salmon fillets (3 ounces)
- 2 teaspoons garlic salt
- 3 teaspoons chopped fresh cilantro

DIRECTIONS

In a bowl, mix the balsamic vinegar and olive oil.
Rub the garlic over the fillets, then pour over the oil and vinegar.
Place salmon fillets in an ovenproof dish and season with basil, cilantro, and garlic salt. Marinate for 25 minutes.
Preheat the oven rack, place the salmon, and bake for about 15 minutes, turning on both sides.
Serve.

NUTRITION:
Per Serving: Calories 391 | Protein 15g | Carbohydrates 4g

BEANS SALAD

COOKING: 0 min **PREPARATION: 5 min** **SERVES: 10**

INGREDIENTS

- 2 tablespoons chopped fresh parsley, or to taste
- ¼ cup olive oil
- 1 15-ounce can of dark red beans, rinsed and drained
- ½ onion, chopped
- 15 ounces cannellini beans, rinsed and drained
- 2 cloves garlic, minced
- 1 15-ounce can of chickpeas, rinsed and drained
- salt and ground black pepper to taste
- 1 lemon, squeezed

DIRECTIONS

Combine the chickpeas, cannellini beans, and garbanzo beans in a bowl.

Add lemon juice, onion, olive oil, garlic, parsley, salt, and black pepper and mix well.

Serve.

NUTRITION:

Per Serving: Calories 193 | Protein 7g | Carbohydrates 25g

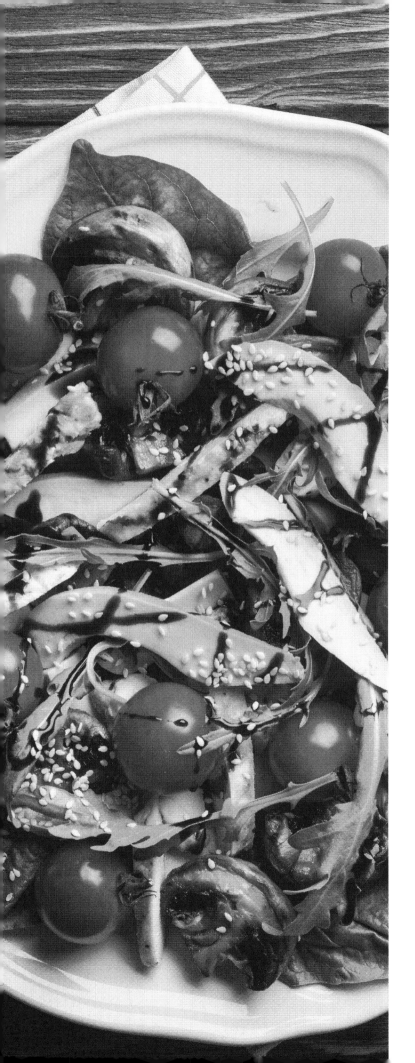

DINNER RECIPES

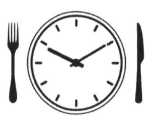

CLASSIC HUMMUS

COOKING: 0 min **PREPARATION: 5 min** **SERVES: 15**

INGREDIENTS

- 1 ½ teaspoons tahini
- ¾ teaspoon salt
- black pepper to taste
- 1 tablespoon and ½ teaspoon olive oil
- 1 ½ cloves garlic, divided
- ¾ (19 ounces) can of chickpeas, half the liquid reserved
- 3 tablespoons lemon juice

DIRECTIONS

In a blender, mince the garlic. Pour the chickpeas into the blender, saving about 1 tablespoon for the garnish. Add the reserved liquid, tahini, salt, and lemon juice to the blender. Blend until creamy and smooth.

Transfer the mixture to a medium bowl.

Sprinkle with pepper and drizzle olive oil on top. Garnish with the reserved chickpeas.

NUTRITION:

Per Serving: Calories 60 | Protein 2g | Carbohydrates 22g

CLASSIC TOFU STEW

COOKING: 12 min **PREPARATION: 5 min** **SERVES: 2**

INGREDIENTS

- 1 tablespoon olive oil
- 6 ounces extra-fine tofu, pressed and crumbled
- 1 cup spinach
- Sea salt and ground black pepper to taste
- 1/2 teaspoon turmeric powder
- 1/4 teaspoon cumin powder
- 1/2 teaspoon garlic powder
- 1 handful fresh chives, chopped

DIRECTIONS

In a skillet over medium heat, heat the olive oil. When hot, add the tofu and cook for 10 minutes, stirring.

Add spinach and herbs and continue to cook for another 2 minutes.

Garnish with fresh chives and serve hot. Enjoy!

NUTRITION:

Per Serving: Calories: 202 | Protein: 14g | Carbohydrates: 7g

TRADITIONAL SPANISH TORTILLA

COOKING: 20 min — **PREPARATION: 5 min** — **SERVES: 2**

INGREDIENTS

- 3 tablespoons olive oil
- 2 medium potatoes, peeled and diced
- 1/2 white onion, chopped
- 8 tablespoons gram flour
- 8 tablespoons water
- Sea salt and ground black pepper for seasoning
- 1/2 teaspoon Spanish paprika

DIRECTIONS

Heat 2 tablespoons olive oil in a skillet over medium heat. Add the onion and let it wilt; next, add the potatoes and cook for 15 minutes.

In a bowl, mix the paprika, water, flour, salt, and black pepper.

Add the potato and onion mixture.

Heat 1 tablespoon olive oil in the same skillet. Pour 1/2 of the batter into the skillet. Cook the tortilla for about 10 minutes.

Repeat the process with the remaining batter and serve warm.

NUTRITION:
Per Serving: Calories: 379 | Protein: 5g | Carbohydrates 46g

MEXICAN STYLE OMELETTE

COOKING: 10 min — **PREPARATION: 5 min** — **SERVES: 2**

INGREDIENTS

- 2 tablespoons olive oil
- Kala namak salt and ground black pepper
- 1 small onion, chopped
- 2 Spanish peppers, seeded and chopped
- 1/2 cup chickpea flour
- 1/2 teaspoon dried Mexican oregano
- 1/2 cup water
- 3 tablespoons unsweetened rice milk
- 2 tablespoons nutritional yeast
- 1/4 cup of salsa

DIRECTIONS

In a skillet heat olive oil over medium-high heat. Once hot, sauté the onion and peppers until tender.

Mix the chickpea flour with the water, yeast, milk, oregano, salt, and black pepper. Then, pour the mixture into the skillet. Cook for about 5 minutes per side.

Serve with the sauce and enjoy!

NUTRITION:
Per Serving: Calories: 329 | Protein: 12g | Carbohydrates: 35g

TASTY TAPENADE

COOKING: 0 min   **PREPARATION: 2 min**   **SERVES: 6**

INGREDIENTS

- 2 ¾ tablespoons chopped fresh parsley
- 1 tablespoon and 1 ½ teaspoon lemon juice
- 2 ¼ cloves garlic, peeled
- ¾ cup pitted kalamata olives
- 1 tablespoon and ½ teaspoon olive oil
- salt and pepper to taste
- 1 tablespoon and ½ teaspoon capers

DIRECTIONS

Place the garlic cloves in a blender or food processor and mince. Add the capers, olives, lemon juice, parsley, and olive oil. Season to taste with salt and pepper.

NUTRITION:
Per Serving: Calories 90 | Protein 1g | Carbohydrates 2g

THE SIMPLEST TAHINI SAUCE

COOKING: 0 min   **PREPARATION: 1 min**   **SERVES: 10**

INGREDIENTS

- ⅔ cup and 1 tablespoon tahini
- ¼ cup and 1 teaspoon and ⅓ teaspoon honey, or more to taste
- ¾ teaspoon and ☐ teaspoon ground cinnamon

DIRECTIONS

Combine honey, cinnamon, and tahini, in a bowl. Stir until well combined.

NUTRITION:
Per Serving: Calories 20 | Protein 1g | Carbohydrates 1g

RAINBOW CHARD RECIPE

COOKING: 20 min | **PREPARATION: 5 min** | **SERVES: 4**

INGREDIENTS

- 1 cup arugula
- 4 cloves garlic, minced
- 8 eggs, beaten
- 1 cup shredded cheddar cheese
- Salt and ground black pepper to taste
- 2 tablespoons olive oil
- ½ cup chopped rainbow chard
- 2 cups fresh spinach

DIRECTIONS

1. In a skillet, heat oil over medium heat. Sauté spinach, chard, and arugula until tender, about 5 minutes.
2. Add garlic, cook and stir until fragrant, about 3-4 minutes.
3. Mix eggs and cheese in a bowl; pour into chard mixture. Cover and cook for about 7 minutes. Season with salt and pepper.

NUTRITION:
Per Serving: Calories 208 | Protein 8g | Carbohydrates 48g

CAPRESE TOAST

COOKING: 5 min | **PREPARATION: 5 min** | **SERVES: 10**

INGREDIENTS

- 3 tablespoons and ☐ teaspoon fresh basil leaves
- 2.14 large tomatoes, sliced 1/4 inch thick
- 2 tablespoons and ☐ teaspoon extra virgin olive oil
- salt and ground black pepper to taste
- 10 slices of sourdough bread
- 1.43 cloves of garlic, peeled
- 7 pounds fresh mozzarella cheese, cut into 1/4-inch thick slices

DIRECTIONS

Toast the bread slices and rub one side of each slice with garlic. Place a slice of mozzarella, a few basil leaves to taste, and a slice of tomato on each piece of toasted bread. Drizzle with olive oil, salt, and black pepper.

NUTRITION:
Per Serving: Calories 190 | Protein 11g | Carbohydrates 33g

PORK CHOPS

COOKING: 15 min   **PREPARATION: 10 min**   **SERVES: 6**

INGREDIENTS

- 6 pork chops with bone
- 1 tablespoon dried sage, crumbled
- 1 ½ bay leaves, crumbled
- 1 tablespoon dried rosemary leaves, crumbled
- ¾ teaspoon white sugar
- 2 teaspoons salt
- 1 ½ teaspoons dried thyme
- ½ cup extra-virgin olive oil
- 1 ½ teaspoon fennel seeds, crushed

DIRECTIONS

Mix and combine the thyme, rosemary, sage, bay leaf, sugar, fennel seeds, and salt in a bowl.

Top the pork chops with the herb mixture you created and drizzle with olive oil. Refrigerate for 1 hour.

Lightly oil a grill and preheat.

Grill the chops until golden brown, about 6 minutes per side. Serve warm.

NUTRITION:

Per Serving: Calories 389 | Protein 9g | Carbohydrates 2g

GREEK TAHINI SAUCE

COOKING: 0 min   **PREPARATION: 5 min**   **SERVES: 12**

INGREDIENTS

- salt and ground black pepper to taste
- 1 tablespoon chopped fresh parsley
- 2 teaspoons minced garlic, or to taste
- ½ cup regular yogurt
- ½ cup tahini
- 2 tablespoons lemon juice
- 1 cup water, or more if needed
- 1 teaspoon vinegar
- 1 tablespoon olive oil

DIRECTIONS

In a bowl, combine the yogurt, water, lemon juice, tahini, garlic, vinegar, olive oil, salt, pepper and, parsley.

Whisk until the mixture is smooth.

NUTRITION:

Per Serving: Calories 77 | Protein 4g | Carbohydrates 5g

MARINADE FOR EVERY DISH

COOKING: 0 min   **PREPARATION: 5 min**   **SERVES: 2**

INGREDIENTS

- 2 ½ cloves garlic, crushed
- 1 lemon, squeezed
- ¼ cup red wine vinegar
- ½ teaspoon garlic powder
- ground black pepper to taste
- ½ teaspoon dried sage
- ½ teaspoon dried thyme
- ½ teaspoon dried rosemary
- ½ teaspoon dried basil
- ½ teaspoon dried oregano
- ½ teaspoon dried marjoram

DIRECTIONS

Combine garlic, lemon juice, olive oil, rosemary, thyme, vinegar, sage, marjoram, garlic powder, basil, pepper, and oregano in a large shallow dish.

Stir with a fork until the mixture appears uniform.

NUTRITION:

Per Serving: Calories 393 | Protein 2g | Carbohydrates 11g

SIMPLE SALMON SOUP

COOKING: 15 min   **PREPARATION: 5 min**   **SERVES: 6**

INGREDIENTS

- 2 pounds of potatoes cut into rounds
- 4 onions, chopped
- Black pepper
- juice of 1 lemon
- 1 green bell pepper, chopped
- Extra virgin olive oil
- 1/2 teaspoon dried oregano
- 2 oz fresh dill, divided, chopped
- 1 teaspoon ground cumin
- ¾ teaspoon ground cilantro
- 2 carrots, cut into rounds
- 2 lbs salmon fillet
- Salt
- 6 cups chicken broth
- 1 teaspoon ground cumin

DIRECTIONS

In a saucepan, heat 2 tablespoons of extra virgin olive oil. Cook for about 4 minutes over medium heat, adding the bell pepper, onions, and garlic, stirring often.

Add some dill, stir for another 50 seconds.

Add carrots, broth, potatoes, spices, and season with pepper and salt.

Bring to a boil, then lower heat and continue to cook for 6 minutes.

Season the salmon with salt and add it to the boiling pot of soup. Cook for 3 minutes.

Add the dill, lemon zest, and lemon juice while stirring.

Serve immediately.

NUTRITION:

Per Serving: Calories 203 | Protein 19g | Carbohydrates 15g

MUSSEL STEW

COOKING: 25 min **PREPARATION: 10 min** **SERVES: 12**

INGREDIENTS

- ⅔ pound broccoli, thick stalks peeled
- 1 cup teaspoon olive oil
- pounds potatoes, peeled and diced
- 2 tablespoons chopped fresh parsley
- anchovy fillets, rinsed and chopped
- salt to taste
- 3 pounds mussels, cleaned and peeled
- 1 cup water
- cloves garlic, minced

DIRECTIONS

Place the potatoes in a saucepan along with the cold water and salt.
Bring to a boil and cook for about 10-15 minutes, then drain.
In another pot, bring the water to a boil and add the salt.
Put in the broccoli and cook. Drain and cut into lengths of about 2 inches.
In a skillet, combine the garlic, crushed anchovies, and oil. Cook over high heat for 2 minutes.
Combine the mussels in the skillet and add broccoli, parsley, the potatoes.
Add 1 cup of water and season with salt. Cook until the mussels are open. Serve immediately.

NUTRITION:
Per Serving: Calories 199 | Protein 7g | Carbohydrates 19g

BULGUR WITH SPINACH AND TOMATOES

COOKING: 15 min **PREPARATION: 5 min** **SERVES: 6**

INGREDIENTS

- 2 cups bulgur
- 1/2 teaspoon ground cumin
- 1/4 teaspoon salt
- 3 cups water
- 15 ounces rinsed chickpeas or beans
- 7 ounces fresh spinach
- 2 cups cherry tomatoes
- 1 small red onion, halved and thinly sliced
- 1 cup crumbled feta cheese
- 1/4 cup hummus
- 2 tablespoons chopped fresh mint
- 3 tablespoons lemon juice

DIRECTIONS

In a saucepan, place the water, salt, bulgur, and ground cumin, bringing to a boil. Cook for 15 minutes over low heat, covered. Stir in chickpea beans.
Remove from heat, add spinach, and stir. Let stand for about 5 minutes. Stir in the remaining ingredients.
Serve hot or cold to your liking.

NUTRITION:
Per Serving: Calories 106 | Protein 16g | Carbohydrates 6g

PATTIES KALE SALAD

COOKING: 30 min   **PREPARATION: 10 min**   **SERVES: 8**

INGREDIENTS

- 2 teaspoons chopped parsley
- 1 cup sour cream or regular yogurt
- 1/2 cup milk
- 1 package of legume patties
- 1/2 teaspoon salt
- 3 cups torn kale
- 1/2 cup of peeled cucumber with chopped seeds
- 3 cups fresh spinach
- 4 large hard-boiled eggs, chopped
- 1 medium ripe avocado, finely chopped
- 1 cup crumbled feta cheese
- 1 cup pitted olives, finely chopped
- 3 medium tomatoes, seeded and finely chopped
- 9 strips of bacon, cooked and crumbled

DIRECTIONS

Prepare and cook the legume patties.
Let cool and crumble or coarsely chop.
In a bowl, mix milk, parsley, sour cream, cucumber, and salt.
In another bowl, combine the kale and spinach and then arrange on a plate.
Place crumbled meatballs and remaining ingredients on top.
Drizzle with dressing

NUTRITION:
Per Serving: Calories 258 | Protein 13g | Carbohydrates 16g

CHICKEN MEATBALLS

COOKING: 10 min   **PREPARATION: 5 min**   **SERVES: 2**

INGREDIENTS

- 1/2 cup chicken
- 2 tsp salt
- 2 tbsp parsley
- 2 tbsp olive oil

DIRECTIONS

Chop the chicken breast and place it in a bowl.
Boil the potatoes and mash them with a fork.
Mix everything with chopped parsley and salt.
Form patties and cook them in a pan with 2 tablespoons of oil.
Enjoy!

NUTRITION:
Per Serving: Calories 254 | Protein 14g | Carbohydrates 29g

HUMMUS OF CAULIFLOWER AND AVOCADO

COOKING: 20 min **PREPARATION: 5 min** **SERVES: 2**

INGREDIENTS

- 1 medium cauliflower, stalkless and chopped
- 1 large avocado, peeled, pitted, and chopped
- ¼ cup extra virgin olive oil
- 2 garlic cloves
- ½ tablespoon lemon juice
- ½ tablespoon onion powder
- Sea salt and ground black pepper to taste
- ¼ cup fresh coriander, chopped
- 2 carrots

DIRECTIONS

Preheat the oven to 450°F and line a baking sheet with aluminum foil.

Place the chopped cauliflower on the baking sheet and drizzle with 2 tablespoons of olive oil.

Roast the cauliflower in the oven for 20 minutes.

Remove the tray from the oven and leave the cauliflower to cool.

Add the cauliflower, avocado, oil, lemon juice, onion, salt and pepper, and coriander to a food processor. Blend until it becomes smooth hummus.

Transfer hummus to a medium-sized bowl, cover let sit in the fridge for 20 minutes.

Cut the carrots into slices and enjoy with the hummus!

NUTRITION:

Per Serving: Calories 416 | Protein 3g | Carbohydrates 8g

QUICK PINTO BEAN SOUP WITH HERBS

COOKING: 10 min **PREPARATION: 5 min** **SERVES: 5**

INGREDIENTS

- 2 cups precooked beans
- 3 tablespoons olive oil
- 1 large onion, chopped
- 1 celery with leaves, chopped
- 1 bell bell pepper, seeded and chopped
- 1 red chili pepper, seeded and chopped
- 1 teaspoon garlic, minced
- 1 teaspoon dried thyme
- 1 teaspoon dried marjoram
- 1 teaspoon dried oregano
- 1 cup tomatoes, pureed
- 4 cups vegetable broth
- Sea salt and ground black pepper, to taste
- 1 bay leaf

DIRECTIONS

In a saucepan, heat olive oil over medium heat. Once hot, sauté the onion, celery, and peppers for about 2 minutes.

Sauté the garlic and herbs for about 2 minutes.

Add the vegetable broth, salt, black pepper, bay leaf, and the precooked beans.

NUTRITION:

Per Serving: Calories: 409 | Protein: 21 | Carbohydrates: 56g

CARROT FAKE MEATBALLS

COOKING: 0 min   **PREPARATION: 10 min**   **SERVES: 8**

INGREDIENTS

- 1 large, grated carrot
- 1 ½ cups old-fashioned oats
- 1 cup raisins
- 1 cup dates
- 1 cup coconut flakes
- 1/4 teaspoon ground cloves
- 1/2 teaspoon ground cinnamon

DIRECTIONS

In your food processor, place carrot, oats, raisins, dates, coconut flakes, cloves and cinnamon and blend until a mixture forms.
Form the batter into equal balls.
Place in refrigerator for 15 minutes.
Enjoy!

NUTRITION:

Per Serving: Calories: 395 | Protein: 22g | Carbohydrates: 58g

DELICIOUS CRISPY SWEET POTATOES

COOKING: 20 min   **PREPARATION: 5 min**   **SERVES: 4**

INGREDIENTS

- 4 sweet potatoes, peeled and grated
- 2 eggs
- 1/4 cup nutritional yeast
- 2 tablespoons tahini
- 2 tablespoons chickpea flour
- 1 teaspoon shallot powder
- 1 teaspoon garlic powder
- 1 teaspoon paprika
- Sea salt and ground black pepper, to taste

DIRECTIONS

Begin by preheating the oven to 380 degrees F. Line a baking sheet with baking paper.
Mix the potatoes, eggs, tahini sauce, and all spices.
Form into balls and bake them for 20 minutes.
Enjoy!

NUTRITION:

Per Serving: Calories: 215 | Protein: 8g | Carbohydrates: 35g

GLAZED CARROTS – SIDE DISH

COOKING: 20 min **PREPARATION:** 5 min **SERVES:** 6

INGREDIENTS

- 2 pounds of baby carrots
- 1/4 cup olive oil
- 1/4 cup apple cider vinegar
- 1/2 teaspoon red pepper flakes
- Sea salt and freshly ground black pepper, to taste
- 1 tablespoon agave syrup
- 2 tablespoons soy sauce
- 1 tablespoon fresh cilantro, chopped

DIRECTIONS

Preheating the oven to 380 degrees F.

Then, in a bowl mix agave syrup, olive oil, red pepper, vinegar, salt, black pepper, and soy sauce. Add carrots and mix again.

Bake carrots for 20 minutes; garnish with cilantro when done.

NUTRITION:
Per Serving: Calories: 165 | Protein: 2g | Carbohydrates: 16g

---

GARLIC CROUTONS

COOKING: 0 min **PREPARATION:** 10 min **SERVES:** 4

INGREDIENTS

- 1 whole-wheat baguette, sliced
- 4 tablespoons extra virgin olive oil
- 1/2 teaspoon sea salt
- 3 garlic cloves, cut in half

DIRECTIONS

In a skillet, toast the bread slices. Next, brush each bread slice with olive oil and sprinkle with sea salt. Rub the garlic on each slice.

NUTRITION:
Per Serving: Calories: 289 | Protein: 9g | Carbohydrates: 44g

QUICK ZUCCHINI ROLLS

COOKING: 0 min | **PREPARATION: 10 min** | **SERVES: 5**

INGREDIENTS

- 1 cup hummus, preferably homemade
- 1 medium tomato, chopped
- 1 teaspoon mustard
- 1/4 teaspoon oregano
- 1/2 teaspoon cayenne pepper
- Sea salt and ground black pepper, to taste
- 1 large zucchini, cut into strips
- 2 tablespoons fresh basil, chopped
- 2 tablespoons fresh parsley, chopped

DIRECTIONS

In a bowl, mix the mustard, tomato, hummus, oregano, cayenne pepper, salt and black pepper.

Divide the filling among the zucchini strips and distribute evenly. Roll up zucchini and garnish with fresh basil and parsley.

NUTRITION:

Per Serving: Calories: 99 | Protein: 3g | Carbohydrates: 12g

BEANS DRESSING

COOKING: 0 min | **PREPARATION: 10 min** | **SERVES: 6**

INGREDIENTS

- 10 ounces canned cannellini beans, drained
- 1 garlic clove, minced
- 2 roasted peppers, sliced
- Freshly ground black pepper, to taste
- 1/2 teaspoon ground cumin
- 1/2 teaspoon mustard seeds
- 1/2 teaspoon ground bay leaf
- 3 tablespoons tahini
- 2 tablespoons fresh Italian parsley, chopped

DIRECTIONS

Place the beans, garlic, peppers, pepper, cumin, mustard seeds, bay leaf, and tahini in a blender, and blend.

Transfer sauce to a serving bowl and garnish with fresh parsley.

Serve with pita wedges, tortilla chips or vegetable sticks, if desired.

NUTRITION:

Per Serving: Calories: 123 | Protein: 5g | Carbohydrates: 15g

ROASTED CHICKPEA SNACK

COOKING: **PREPARATION:** 30 min   **SERVES:** 8

INGREDIENTS

- 1 cup roasted chickpeas, drained
- 2 tablespoons coconut oil, melted
- 1/4 cup raw pumpkin seeds
- 1/4 cup raw pecan halves
- 1/3 cup dried cherries

DIRECTIONS

Preheat oven to 375 degrees F.
Mix the chickpeas with coconut oil.
Cook the chickpeas in the oven for 15 minutes, turning occasionally.
Mix the chickpeas with the pumpkin seeds and pecan halves. Continue baking until the nuts are fragrant, about 10 minutes; let cool completely.
Add the dried cherries and stir to combine.

NUTRITION:
Per Serving: Calories: 109 | Protein: 3g | Carbohydrates: 7g

HEALTHY ZUCCHINI ROLLS

COOKING: **PREPARATION:** 10 min   **SERVES:** 5

INGREDIENTS

- 1 cup rice
- 1 carrot, grated
- 1 small onion, grated
- 1 avocado, chopped
- 1 garlic clove, minced
- Sea salt and ground black pepper, to taste
- 1 medium zucchini, cut into strips

DIRECTIONS

Bring rice to a boil and cover with a lid; cook for 12 minutes. In a bowl, mix rice, carrot, onion, avocado, garlic, salt and black pepper.
Divide the filling among the zucchini strips and distribute evenly. Roll the zucchini and serve with a sauce of your choice.

NUTRITION:
Per Serving: Calories: 129 | Protein: 2g | Carbohydrates: 15g

HUMMUS WITH TOMATOES

COOKING: **PREPARATION:** 10 min **SERVES:** 8

INGREDIENTS

- 1/2 cup hummus
- 2 tablespoons vegan mayonnaise
- 1/4 cup shallots
- 16 cherry tomatoes
- 2 tablespoons fresh cilantro

DIRECTIONS

Chop the shallots and cilantro on a cutting board. Scoop out the pulp from the tomatoes.

In a bowl, mix the hummus, shallots, tomato pulp and mayonnaise.

Divide the mixture among the tomatoes. Garnish with cilantro.

NUTRITION:

Per Serving: Calories: 49 | Protein: 1g | Carbohydrates: 4g

SEAFOOD SOUP

COOKING: 30 min **PREPARATION:** 10 min **SERVES:** 6

INGREDIENTS

- 1½ lbs salmon, boneless fillets or other firm fish, pin bones removed, fillets cut into 1" pieces
- 2¾ cups baby spinach
- 1½ cups clam juice
- 2¼ cups heavy whipping cream
- 3 tsp dried sage or dried thyme
- 12 oz. shrimp peeled and deveined
- ¾ cup cream cheese
- salt and ground black pepper
- ¾ tbsp red chili peppers
- 2 cups celery stalks, sliced
- ¾ lemon, juice and zest
- fresh sage, optional for garnish
- 6 tbsp butter
- 3 garlic cloves, minced

DIRECTIONS

Melt the butter in a saucepan over medium heat.

Add the garlic and celery and cook for 5 minutes, stirring occasionally.

Add the cream, clam juice, sage, cream cheese, and lemon juice, and zest.

Allow simmering for 10 minutes without a lid.

Add the shrimp and fish.

Simmer until the fish is just cooked through.

Add the spinach and stir until wilted.

Season with salt and pepper to taste.

Before serving for extra flavor, garnish with red pepper and sage.

NUTRITION:

Per Serving: Calories 257 | Protein 21g | Carbohydrates 12g

SALAD IN A JAR

COOKING: **PREPARATION:** 10 min   **SERVES:** 3

INGREDIENTS

- ¾ oz. scallions, sliced
- 3 oz. red bell peppers
- 3 oz. cherry tomatoes
- 3 carrots
- 12 oz. smoked salmon or rotisserie chicken
- 1½ cups leafy greens
- ¾ cup vegan mayonnaise or olive oil
- 3 avocados

DIRECTIONS

Shred the vegetables.
Initially, place the vegetables in the bottom of the jar.
Add carrot, avocado, scallion, tomato and peppers in layers.
Add the grilled chicken or smoked salmon.
Just before serving, put a little mayonnaise.

NUTRITION:
Per Serving: Calories 401 | Protein 23g | Carbohydrates 31g

TUNA SALAD WITH CAPERS

COOKING: **PREPARATION:** 8-10 min   **SERVES:** 2

INGREDIENTS

- ½ tbsp capers
- 2 oz. tuna in olive oil
- ¾ oz. leek, finely chopped
- salt and pepper
- ¼ cup mayonnaise or vegan mayonnaise
- ¼ tsp chili flakes
- 1 tbsp crème fraîche or cream cheese

DIRECTIONS

Allow the tuna to drain.
Season with salt, pepper and red pepper flakes.
Mix all ingredients together.

NUTRITION:
Per Serving: Calories 271 | Protein 23g | Carbohydrates 25g

EASY TUNA ZOODLE SALAD

COOKING: 15 **PREPARATION: 20** **SERVES: 6**

INGREDIENTS

- 6 eggs
- 1½ cups tomatoes diced
- 2 lbs zucchini
- 3 tsp onion powder
- 23 oz. canned tuna in water drained
- 1¼ cups mayonnaise
- ground black pepper and salt

DIRECTIONS

In a pot of boiling water, place the eggs.
To facilitate peeling, add a little salt to the water.
For soft-boiled eggs, cook 5-6 minutes, for medium eggs 6-8 minutes, and for hard-boiled eggs 8-10 minutes.
To cool the eggs, place them in a bowl of ice-cold water.
Peel the eggs and cut them in half.
In bowl, mix the tuna, mayonnaise and onion.
Add salt and pepper to taste.
Using a potato peeler, make thin strips of zucchini or, with a spiralizer, create zucchini spirals.
Place zoodles in a bowl along with olive oil, salt, and pepper to taste.
Place the zoodles on plates and add the tuna, eggs, and diced tomatoes.

NUTRITION:

Per Serving: Calories 375 | Protein 24g | Carbohydrates 31g

GREEN BEANS AND GROUND BEEF

COOKING: 15-20 min **PREPARATION: 5 min** **SERVES: 4**

INGREDIENTS

- 25 oz. ground beef or ground turkey
- 7 oz. butter
- salt and pepper
- 18 oz. fresh green beans
- 2/3 cup mayonnaise

DIRECTIONS

In a bowl, rinse and cut green beans.
In a large skillet, heat the butter.
Cook ground beef over high heat until almost done.
Add pepper and salt to taste and lower the heat a bit.
In the same skillet, add the butter and fry the green beans for 5-6 minutes, occasionally stir in the ground beef.
Season the beans with salt and pepper as well.
Add mayonnaise and serve with butter.

NUTRITION:

Per Serving: Calories 245 | Protein 17g | Carbohydrates 14g

BACON CHEESEBURGER WRAPS

COOKING: 25 min **PREPARATION:** 5-7 min **SERVES:** 4

INGREDIENTS

- 7 oz. bacon
- ½ tsp salt
- ¼ tsp pepper
- 4 oz. mushrooms sliced
- 1 cup shredded cheddar cheese
- 8 cherry tomatoes sliced
- 1½ lbs ground beef or ground turkey
- 1 butterhead lettuce with leaves separated and washed

DIRECTIONS

In a skillet, cook the bacon over medium heat for about 10-15 minutes.

When it becomes crispy, remove the bacon from the skillet and set it aside.

Sauté the mushrooms in the bacon fat, over medium-high heat, for about 5 minutes.

When browned and tender, set aside.

Add the ground beef, salt and pepper.

Sauté the beef for about 10 minutes breaking up any pieces for about 8-10 minutes until evenly browned.

Before serving, pour ground beef over lettuce leaves and place cheddar cheese, mushrooms, tomatoes and bacon on top.

NUTRITION:

Per Serving: Calories 436 | Protein 24g | Carbohydrates 22g

MUSHROOM CAULIFLOWER RISOTTO

COOKING: 30-35 min **PREPARATION:** 15-20 min **SERVES:** 6

INGREDIENTS

- 3 garlic cloves
- 1½ large cauliflower
- 1½ shallots
- 1½ cups vegetable stock
- 1½ cups heavy whipping cream
- 1¼ cups white wine
- 14 oz. mushrooms
- salt and pepper
- ¾ cup shredded Parmesan cheese
- 6 oz. butter
- fresh thyme

DIRECTIONS

Bring the broth to a boil over medium-high heat.

Shred the mushrooms and fry them in butter.

Finely chop the shallot and garlic and then add them to the mushrooms.

Add the grated cauliflower to a pan.

Add the broth and half of the wine.

Let simmer without the lid on until the liquid begins to boil, then pour off the remaining wine.

Simmer, add the cream until the cauliflower is soft and most of the liquid has disappeared.

Stir in Parmesan cheese and add fresh thyme before serving.

NUTRITION:

Per Serving: Calories 455 | Protein 9g | Carbohydrates 54g

ITALIAN STYLE OMELETTE

COOKING: 30 min **PREPARATION: 9-10 min** **SERVES: 2**

INGREDIENTS

- 4 oz. (3 2/3 cups) fresh spinach
- 4 eggs
- 2½ oz. diced bacon or chorizo
- ½ cup heavy whipping cream
- 2½ oz. (2/3 cup) cheddar cheese, shredded
- salt and pepper
- 1 tbsp butter

DIRECTIONS

Preheat the oven to 350°F (175°C).
Use ramekins or grease on a baking sheet.
In a skillet over medium heat, sauté bacon in butter until crispy. Insert the spinach and stir until wilted.
Set the skillet aside.
Mix eggs with cream and pour into ramekins or a baking dish.
Add spinach, bacon, and cheese on top and place in the center of the oven.
Place in the oven for 30 minutes or until golden brown on top.

NUTRITION:
Per Serving: Calories 320 | Protein 11g | Carbohydrates 25g

SALMON WITH CHIVES AND SCRAMBLED EGGS

COOKING: 15 min **PREPARATION: 5 min** **SERVES: 4**

INGREDIENTS

- 8 eggs
- 4 tbsp fresh chives, chopped
- 8 oz. cured salmon
- 1 cup heavy whipping cream
- 8 tbsp butter
- salt and pepper

DIRECTIONS

Crack and beat the eggs well.
In a skillet, melt the butter and then stir together with the eggs. Add the cream to the mixture and heat carefully while stirring.
Over low heat, let the mixture simmer for a few minutes, constantly stirring to make the eggs smooth.
Season with chopped chives, salt and pepper.
Serve with slices of salmon.

NUTRITION:
Per Serving: Calories 411 | Protein 26g | Carbohydrates 49g

SMOKED SALMON WITH AVOCADO

COOKING: **PREPARATION:** 5 min   **SERVES:** 6

INGREDIENTS

- 6 (2 2/3 lbs) avocados
- 25 oz. smoked salmon
- salt and pepper
- 6 tbsp mayonnaise

DIRECTIONS

Open the avocado in half and remove the stone.
Using a spoon, scoop out the avocado pieces and place them on a plate.
Toss together the mayonnaise and salmon on the plate.
Top with black pepper and a pinch of sea salt.

NUTRITION:
Per Serving: Calories 487 | Protein 22g | Carbohydrates 34g

PAPRIKA CHICKEN WITH RUTABAGA

COOKING: 35 min   **PREPARATION:** 15 min   **SERVES:** 2

INGREDIENTS

- 1 lb rutabaga or celery root, peeled and cut into 2" (5 cm) pieces
- ½ tbsp paprika powder
- 1 lb chicken thighs (bone-in with skin) or chicken drumsticks
- 1 tbsp olive oil
- salt and pepper
- Garlic and paprika mayo
- ½ tsp paprika powder
- ½ tsp garlic powder
- 2/5 cup mayonnaise or vegan mayonnaise
- salt and pepper

DIRECTIONS

Preheat the oven to 400°F (200°C).
In a baking dish, place the rutabaga and chicken.
Season with paprika powder, salt and pepper. Add a few drops of olive oil and mix sufficiently.
Bake for 35 minutes or until chicken is well cooked. When the chicken is almost cooked, or the rutabaga is getting too golden brown lower the heat.
Mix the mayonnaise with the dressing.
Serve along with the roasted chicken and rutabaga.

NUTRITION:
Per Serving: Calories 366 | Protein 19g | Carbohydrates 33g

GINGER LIME CHICKEN

COOKING: 15-20 min **PREPARATION:** 10 min **SERVES:** 6

INGREDIENTS
- 2/5 cup tamari soy sauce or coconut aminos
- 2¼ lbs chicken breasts
- 1½ tsp sesame seeds, toasted, for garnish
- 1½ tbsp fresh cilantro, chopped, for garnish
- 1½ tsp fresh ginger, grated
- 3 tbsp fresh lime juice
- 3 tsp toasted sesame oil
- 1½ pinches chili flakes, extra for garnish
- 1½ tsp lime zest

DIRECTIONS
In a bowl, place the chicken breasts.
So that the chicken can absorb the marinade, prick the chicken using a fork.
In a small bowl, combine the soy sauce, red pepper flakes, sesame oil, lime zest, lime juice, ginger and mix.
Sprinkle the chicken with the resulting mixture and let it marinate in the refrigerator for 2 to 24 hours.
Over medium-high heat a grill pan.
When the pan is ready and hot, insert the chicken, sprinkling it with the marinade.
Cook for about 10-15 minutes, turning the chicken until nice and caramelized on the outside and cooked through on the inside.
Before serving, garnish with sesame seeds, red pepper flakes, and cilantro.

NUTRITION:
Per Serving: Calories 237 | Protein 21g | Carbohydrates 35g

SEEDS CRACKERS

COOKING: 35 min **PREPARATION:** 10 min **SERVES:** 15

INGREDIENTS
- 1/6 cup almond flour
- ½ cup boiling water
- ½ tbsp ground psyllium husk powder
- ½ tsp salt
- 1/6 cup sesame seeds
- 1/6 cup unsalted pumpkin seeds
- 1/6 cup flaxseed or chia seeds
- 1/6 cup unsalted sunflower seeds
- 2 tbsp melted coconut oil

DIRECTIONS
Preheat oven to 300°F (150°C).
Mix all the dry ingredients together in a bowl.
Bring the water to a boil and add the boiling water along with the oil.
Combine the ingredients while stirring.
Knead the dough until it forms a ball and has a smooth consistency.
Place baking paper on a baking sheet and place the dough obtained.
To flatten the dough add another paper on top and use a rolling pin to roll out the mixture.
After removing the top paper, bake for about 35 minutes, taking care to check.
Pay close attention towards the end of baking as the seeds will quickly wilt in contact with the heat.
When they are cooked after turning off the oven, leave the crackers to dry inside. Once ready and cooled, break into pieces and spread butter to taste.

NUTRITION:
Per Serving: Calories 60g | Protein 2g | Carbohydrates 25g

EASY HOT DOG

COOKING: 30 min **PREPARATION: 10 min** **SERVES: 15**

INGREDIENTS

- 4½ egg
- 2 cups almond flour
- 3 tsp vinegar
- ½ cup ground psyllium husk powder
- 3 tsp baking powder
- 2 cups boiling water
- 1½ tsp sea salt
- mayonnaise

DIRECTIONS

In a large bowl, combine the dry ingredients.
Preheat the oven to 350°F (175°C).
After boiling the water, add along with the egg whites the vinegar to the bowl, stirring the mixture for about 50 seconds. Do not over-mix the mix; the consistency should not be too smooth.
Using damp hands, form 10 pieces and roll them into hot dog buns. Place the resulting pieces on a baking sheet and leave enough space between them to double in size.
In the preheated oven, bake for about 30 minutes.
Let cool and serve hot dogs and mayonnaise of your choice.

NUTRITION:
Per Serving: Calories 100 | Protein 9g | Carbohydrates 33g

STUFFED MOZZARELLA AND BASIL MEATBALLS

COOKING: 15 min **PREPARATION: 5 min** **SERVES: 10**

INGREDIENTS

- 3¾ lbs ground beef or ground turkey
- 5 tbsp heavy whipping cream
- 10 oz. (2½ cups) shredded mozzarella cheese
- 2½ tsp salt
- 2½ tbsp dried basil
- 5 garlic cloves, minced
- 2/3 tsp ground black pepper

DIRECTIONS

Combine the cream with the ground beef, basil, garlic, salt and black pepper in a bowl. Combine the ingredients well with your hands or the help of a fork.
With damp hands, form into balls. Depending on their size, they will take longer to cook.
Flatten them in your hand and inside the meatball, put a little bit of cheese, wrapping the meat around the cheese.
Bake the meatballs at 350F degrees for 15 minutes.

NUTRITION:
Per Serving: Calories 217 | Protein 17g | Carbohydrates 33g

CHEESY EGGS

COOKING: 15 min   **PREPARATION: 7-10 min**   **SERVES: 4**

INGREDIENTS

- 12 oz. Ground beef or turkey or pork, cook it any way you like.
- 8 eggs
- 2 cups shredded cheese

DIRECTIONS

In a small baking dish, place the already cooked ground beef mixture.
Preheat the oven to 400°F (200°C).
Poke holes with the help of a spoon and open the eggs in them.
Shred in cheese and sprinkle over the ground meat.
Bake for about 8-10 minutes or until eggs are set.
Before serving, allow cooling for a bit.

NUTRITION:
Per Serving: Calories 424 | Protein 11g | Carbs 33g

HAM QUICHE

COOKING: 15 min   **PREPARATION: 10 min**   **SERVES: 3**

INGREDIENTS

- 6 eggs
- 11 ounces of sliced ham
- 2¼ tablespoons chopped fresh chives
- 5¼ ounces mascarpone or cream cheese

DIRECTIONS

Use ramekins that will withstand the heat of the oven.
Preheat oven to 350°F (180°C).
Place inside a single ramekin three slices of ham making sure to cover the sides and bottom.
Mix together the eggs, chives, mascarpone cheese, salt and pepper in a bowl. The mixture should be homogeneous but not smooth.
Finally, pour the egg mixture into the ramekins.
Bake for 15 minutes or until the egg mixture is cooked.
Serve slightly warm.

NUTRITION:
Per Serving: Calories 421 | Protein 17g | Carbs 35g

SCRAMBLED FETA

COOKING: 10 min **PREPARATION:** 5-8 min **SERVES:** 6

INGREDIENTS

- 4½ oz. feta cheese, crumbled
- 12 oz. bacon
- 12 eggs
- 3 garlic cloves, minced
- salt and ground black pepper
- 6 tbsp butter
- 11 cups fresh baby spinach
- 6 tbsp heavy whipping cream

DIRECTIONS

Mix the eggs and cream together in a bowl until smooth.
Heat a skillet over medium-low heat and put the butter in until completely melted.
Place the garlic and spinach together and let cook until the spinach becomes dry.
Sprinkle with salt and pepper.
In the skillet, place the egg mixture. Cook without touching until the edges become firm and dense.
Lift and gently flip the egg using a spatula, allowing the uncooked eggs to cook.
Continue the process of lifting and turning until the eggs are cooked.
When cooked through, sprinkle with feta cheese and serve immediately.

NUTRITION:

Per Serving: Calories 322 | Protein 18g | Carbs 22g

TAPAS

COOKING: **PREPARATION:** 5 min **SERVES:** 5

INGREDIENTS

- 10 oz. prosciutto
- 1¼ cups cheddar cheese
- 2½ oz. red bell peppers
- 2/3 cup mayonnaise
- 5 oz. cucumber
- 10 oz. chorizo

DIRECTIONS

Cut the cheese, prosciutto and vegetables into cubes or sticks.
Arrange on a plate to your liking
Serve and enjoy.

NUTRITION:

Per Serving: Calories 80 | Protein 12g | Carbs 24g

PESTO EGGS MUFFINS

COOKING: 10 min   **PREPARATION:** 5-8 min   **SERVES:** 4

INGREDIENTS

- 8 eggs
- 1 cup shredded cheddar cheese
- 3 1/3 oz. cooked bacon or salami, chopped
- 2/3 oz. scallions, finely chopped
- 1 1/3 tbsp red pesto or green pesto (optional)
- salt and pepper, to taste

DIRECTIONS

In a muffin pan, place ovenproof ramekins, or grease a muffin pan with butter.

Preheat the oven to 350°F (175°C).

Place the cooked bacon, scallions, or salami in the bottom of the baking dish.

Combine together the eggs, pesto, salt and pepper; combine until smooth.

Pour the resulting egg mixture over the meat and scallions. Sprinkle with cheese.

Place in the oven for 15-20 minutes.

Let them cool for 15 minutes and then serve.

NUTRITION:
Per Serving: Calories 211 | Protein 9g | Carbs 10g

HEALTHY GUACAMOLE

COOKING: **PREPARATION:** 10 min   **SERVES:** 8

INGREDIENTS

- 4 ripe avocados
- 2 garlic cloves minced
- 4 tbsp olive oil
- white onion finely chopped
- 1 juice lime
- ½ cup fresh cilantro
- salt and pepper
- tomatoes diced

DIRECTIONS

Open and peel the avocados.

Using a fork, mash them.

Add together and stir in the tomato, onion, olive oil, cilantro, lime juice, and garlic.

Season with salt and pepper to your liking and continue to mix until smooth.

NUTRITION:
Per Serving: Calories 201 | Protein 8g | Carbs 24g

DELICIOUS ROASTED CHICKEN

COOKING: 25-30 min   **PREPARATION: 10 min**   **SERVES: 4**

INGREDIENTS

- 2 lbs chicken legs
- salt and ground black pepper
- 30 oz. broccoli
- 30 oz. cherry tomatoes
- 6 tbsp olive oil
- 3 tbsp Italian seasoning
- Garlic oil
- 3 garlic cloves, pressed
- 6 oz. cononut oil
- salt and ground black pepper

DIRECTIONS

Place the olive oil and seasonings on the chicken thighs.
Preheat the oven to 400°F (200°C).
Place the chicken thighs in a baking dish along with the tomatoes and bake for 40-45 minutes or until the chicken reaches 165 °F (74 °C).
While you're waiting for the chicken to cook, cut off the broccoli florets and slice the stems.
Place the broccoli in a saucepan in the water brought to a boil and add the salt. Drain the water and put the lid on to maintain heat.
In a bowl, combine the ingredients to make the garlic oil and set aside.
Serve the chicken with broccoli, garlic butter, and tomatoes.

NUTRITION:
Per Serving: Calories 225 | Protein 22g | Carbs 26g

MEXICAN SCRAMBLED EGGS

COOKING: 10 min   **PREPARATION: 5 min**   **SERVES: 6**

INGREDIENTS

- 9 eggs
- ¾ oz. scallions finely chopped
- 1¼ cups Pepper Jack cheese shredded
- 3 pickled jalapeños slices finely chopped
- 1½ oz. butter
- 6 oz. tomatoes finely chopped
- salt and pepper

DIRECTIONS

Heat a skillet over medium-high heat and melt the butter inside.
Fry the shallots, tomatoes and jalapeños together for 3-4 minutes.
In a skillet, pour in the beaten eggs.
Stir for 2-4 minutes.
Add the cheese and toppings to your liking.

NUTRITION:
Per Serving: Calories 208 | Protein 12g | Carbs 23g

TASTY PORK WITH FAKE FRIED EGGS

COOKING: 15 min | **PREPARATION: 5-7 min** | **SERVES: 4**

INGREDIENTS
- 8 eggs
- 16 oz. bacon
- 2 oz. frozen cranberries
- 2 tbsp coconut oil
- 2 oz. pecans or walnuts
- 16 oz. kale
- salt and pepper

DIRECTIONS
In a skillet, melt the coconut oil.
Cut the cabbage into large squares.
Quickly cook the cabbage over high heat until the edges are browned.
Remove the cabbage from the pan and set it aside.
In the same skillet, slowly cook the bacon until crispy.
Return the sautéed cabbage to the skillet over low heat and add the walnuts and blueberries.
Combine while stirring until heated through, afterward reserve in a bowl.
Over medium-high heat, cook the eggs in the same skillet used so far. Salt to taste.
For each serving of vegetables, plate two cooked eggs serve immediately.

NUTRITION:
Per Serving: Calories 322 | Protein 12g | Carbs 32g

SAVOURY OVEN PANCAKES

COOKING: 30 min | **PREPARATION: 5 min** | **SERVES: 6**

INGREDIENTS
- 6 eggs
- ¾ cup almond flour
- 3 oz. yellow onion
- 3 tbsp coconut oil
- 5 1/3 oz. turkey or pork bacon
- 1½ tbsp ground psyllium husk powder
- 1½ cups heavy whipping cream
- 1½ tsp baking powder
- ¾ cup cottage cheese
- 1½ tsp salt

DIRECTIONS
Preheat the oven to 350°F (175°C).
In a skillet, heat the coconut oil and add the shredded bacon and onion. Cook until bacon begins to crisp and onion is soft.
Combine eggs, cream, and cottage cheese together in a bowl.
Mix psyllium husk together with almond flour, baking powder, and salt. Whisk until a smooth consistency is achieved.
Let stand for 5 minutes.
In a greased baking dish, pour the pancake batter and sprinkle the top with the bacon and onions.
Bake for 20-25 minutes.

NUTRITION:
Per Serving: Calories 112 | Protein 4g | Carbs 32g

ROLLUPS WITH CHEESE

COOKING: **PREPARATION:** 5 min **SERVES:** 4

INGREDIENTS

- 2 cups cheddar cheese or provolone cheese or Edam cheese, in slices
- 2 oz. Coconut oil

DIRECTIONS

Take a medium to prominent cutting board place the cheese slices to your liking.
Melt the coconut oil.
Sprinkle each cheese slice with the butter and roll up. Quick, serve as a snack.

NUTRITION:
Per Serving: Calories 208 | Protein 7g | Carbs 22g

LEMON SALMON

COOKING: 25 min **PREPARATION:** 10 min **SERVES:** 4

INGREDIENTS

- 4 2/3 oz. butter, thinly & equally sliced divided
- 2/3 lemon, sliced thinly
- 1 1/3 lbs salmon, boneless fillets
- 2/3 tbsp olive oil
- 2/3 tsp sea salt
- 1 1/3 tbsp lemon juice, or juice from 1 lemon
- ground black pepper

DIRECTIONS

Drizzle a baking sheet with olive oil.
Preheat the oven to 400°F (200°C).
Place the salmon in the oiled baking dish, skin side down.
Arrange the lemon slices over the fillets spread a strip of butter.
Bake on the grill for about 25-30 minutes or until the salmon flakes easily.
In a saucepan, heat the remaining part of the butter until it comes to a boil.
When fully cooked, remove from heat and allow to cool. Add lemon juice.
Serve with lemon butter.

NUTRITION:
Per Serving: Calories 211 | Protein 18g | Carbs 21g

GLAZED CHICKEN WINGS

COOKING: 40 min — **PREPARATION: 5 min** — **SERVES: 6**

INGREDIENTS

- 3 tbsp tamari soy sauce
- 2/5 tsp garlic powder
- 2/5 tsp chili flakes
- 2/5 cup coconut aminos
- 2/5 tsp ground ginger
- 3 lbs chicken wings
- 2/5 tsp onion powder

DIRECTIONS

Preheat oven to 450°F (225°C).
On a baking sheet, place the wings with the thickest skin side up. (The wire rack helps the wings cook evenly.)
Bake for about 35 minutes.
Meanwhile, prepare a sauce.
Heat a skillet over medium heat and add the soy sauce, coconut amino acid, and seasonings.
When the sauce begins to simmer, stir. Continue stirring, taking care to adjust the heat to keep it boiling.
The sauce will be ready when it has thickened.
In a large bowl, place the wings and pour the sauce over them.
Take care to evenly cover the wings and serve immediately.

NUTRITION:
Per Serving: Calories 132 | Protein 8g | Carbs 25g

CORN FRITTERS

COOKING: 15 min — **PREPARATION: 10 min** — **SERVES: 2**

INGREDIENTS

- ½ egg
- 1¾ oz. cauliflower cut into florets
- 1 tbsp coconut flour
- ¼ cup coconut oil
- ½ tsp anise seeds or fennel seeds
- 1/8 tsp salt

DIRECTIONS

Finely chop the cauliflower until it looks like flour.
Combine the egg, cauliflower, coconut flour, salt, and anise seeds in a bowl. Mix until a smooth consistency is achieved.
In a skillet over medium heat, heat oil.
Now pour the cauliflower into the pan. I recommend no more than 2 at a time.
Fry for few minutes per side, until golden brown.
Once cooked with the help of a napkin, remove excess oil and serve immediately.

NUTRITION:
Per Serving: Calories 80 | Protein 8g | Carbs 12g

CHEESE WAFFLES

COOKING: 6-8 min **PREPARATION:** 3 min **SERVES:** 4

INGREDIENTS

- 4 eggs
- 4 tbsp almond flour
- 2 cups mozzarella cheese shredded
- 1 oz. butter melted
- 1 pinch salt (optional)

DIRECTIONS

In a bowl, combine all the ingredients and whisk to combine until smooth.

Meanwhile, preheat your waffle maker.

Grease the waffle iron with butter, then pour the mixture evenly onto the waffle iron.

After closing the grill, cook for about 5-7 minutes, depending on your grill.

You can make sure they are cooked by opening the grill.

They will come off quickly if they are cooked through.

Serve with your favorite toppings.

NUTRITION:
Per Serving: Calories 90 | Protein 5g | Carbs 10g

CHEESE OMELET

COOKING: 20 min **PREPARATION:** 10-12 min **SERVES:** 4

INGREDIENTS

- 8 eggs
- 11 oz. green asparagus, into 2.5 cm pieces
- 2 cups baby spinach
- 2 tbsp butter
- 4 oz. goat cheese
- 4 tbsp heavy whipping cream
- 1 scallion, sliced
- salt and pepper

DIRECTIONS

Combine eggs and cream in a bowl until smooth and set aside. Heat butter in a skillet over medium heat until melted. Place the asparagus in the skillet and sauté for about 4 minutes, until crispy. When they are cooked, place them on a plate or bowl but leave the pan's melted butter.

Over low heat, let the pan cool a bit, then pour in the egg mixture. Cook the eggs until the edges are set, then lift the edges and let the melted eggs run underneath to cook.

When fully cooked, sprinkle with salt and pepper to your liking.

Arrange the cooked spinach and asparagus on half of the open omelet.

To finish, sprinkle with cheese with your fingers.

NUTRITION:
Per Serving: Calories 82 | Protein 14g | Carbs 33g

BACON MUSHROOMS DINNER

COOKING: 45 min **PREPARATION: 10-12 min** **SERVES: 2**

INGREDIENTS

- 4 eggs
- 5 oz. bacon, diced
- 3 oz. mushrooms, in quarters
- 1 oz. butter
- ½ tsp onion powder
- salt and pepper
- ½ cup heavy whipping cream
- 2/3 cup shredded cheddar cheese

DIRECTIONS

Preheat the oven to 400°F (200°C).

In a skillet over medium-high heat, melt the butter and then fry the bacon and mushrooms until golden brown—season with salt and pepper to taste.

In a greased baking dish, place the bacon and mushrooms you cooked previously.

In a bowl, place the remaining ingredients and combine. Season with salt and pepper.

Pour the egg mixture over the bacon and mushrooms. Bake in the oven for about 40 minutes.

Tip: If the top of the casserole dish is in danger of burning before fully cooked, cover with aluminum foil.

NUTRITION:
Per Serving: Calories 356 | Protein 5g | Carbs 45g

GREEN CREAMED CABBAGE

COOKING: 20 min **PREPARATION: 5-10 min** **SERVES: 6**

INGREDIENTS

- 2 cups heavy whipping cream
- 3 oz. butter
- 2¼ lbs green cabbage
- 1½ tbsp lemon zest
- ¾ cup fresh parsley finely chopped
- salt and pepper

DIRECTIONS

Shred or slice the cabbage to your liking.

Melt the butter in a skillet over medium-high heat; when the pan is hot, add the cabbage and sauté for a few minutes.

Insert the whipping cream and stir together to combine. Reduce the heat and simmer for 3-5 minutes, or until the cream has a smooth, creamy consistency.

Season with salt and pepper.

Add parsley and lemon zest before serving.

NUTRITION:
Per Serving: Calories 105 | Protein 4g | Carbs 36g

WALNUT AND ZUCCHINI SALAD

COOKING: 20 min **PREPARATION: 5-10 min** **SERVES: 4**

INGREDIENTS

Dressing
- 1 garlic clove finely minced
- ¾ cup mayonnaise or vegan mayonnaise
- 2 tbsp olive oil
- ½ tsp salt
- 2 tsp lemon juice
- ¼ tsp chili powder

Salad:
- 1 head of Romaine lettuce
- 1 cup chopped walnuts or pecans
- ¼ cup finely chopped fresh chives or scallions
- 2 zucchini
- 1 tbsp olive oil
- 4 oz. arugula lettuce
- salt and pepper

DIRECTIONS

Combine In a bowl together with all the ingredients for the dressing.

Cut up the salad. In a bowl, place the arugula, Romaine, and chives.

Open the zucchini, remove the seeds, and cut the zucchini halves into small 1/2 inch pieces.

In a skillet over medium heat, heat the olive oil, then add the zucchini and season with salt and pepper.

Fry until lightly browned without making them soft.

After they are cooked, mix the zucchini into the salad.

In the same pan where you cooked the zucchini, lightly roast the walnuts and season with salt and pepper. Combine the walnuts on the salad and with the dressing.

NUTRITION:
Per Serving: Calories 159 | Protein 7g | Carbs 22g

TORTILLA CHIPS

COOKING: 30 min **PREPARATION: 5-10 min** **SERVES: 4**

INGREDIENTS

- 1 tsp. garlic powder
- 1 tsp. kosher salt
- 2 c. shredded mozzarella
- 1 c. almond flour
- Freshly ground black pepper
- 1/2 tsp. chili powder

DIRECTIONS

Place baking paper on two large baking sheets.

Preheat oven to 350°.

In a bowl, melt the mozzarella cheese in the microwave for about 1 minute and 40 seconds.

Add the garlic powder, almond flour, chili powder, salt, and a little black pepper.

Knead the dough with your hands until it forms a ball.

Place the dough between two sheets of paper and, using a knife cut the dough into triangles.

Place the cut-out triangles on prepared baking sheets and bake for about 12-14 minutes or until edges are golden brown.

NUTRITION:
Per Serving: Calories 45 | Protein 1g | Carbs 2g

INDIAN CREPE

COOKING: 15 min | **PREPARATION: 10 min** | **SERVES: 4**

INGREDIENTS

- 1 cup coconut milk
- 2 tbsp coconut oil, for frying
- 1 tsp ground cumin
- 1 tsp ground coriander seed
- 1 cup almond flour
- salt, to taste
- 1 cup mozzarella cheese, shredded

DIRECTIONS

Place all ingredients in a bowl and mix.
Heat a little oil in a frying pan over low heat. It would be best if you used a non-stick pan.
Pour the batter into the pan until it forms a thin circular shape.
Cook the dosa on low heat for about 3-4 minutes.
When the dosa has turned nice and golden brown, it will be cooked. Fold it over to one side with the help of a spatula.
Serve with coconut chutney.

NUTRITION:
Per Serving: Calories 112 | Protein 2g | Carbs 41g

TASTY BRIAM

COOKING: 90 min | **PREPARATION: 10 min** | **SERVES: 2**

INGREDIENTS

- 3 ripe tomatoes, pureed
- ¼ cup olive oil
- 1 tablespoon chopped fresh parsley
- 1 pound potatoes, peeled and thinly sliced
- sea salt and freshly ground black pepper to taste
- 2 large zucchini, thinly sliced
- 2 small red onions, thinly sliced

DIRECTIONS

Preheat the oven to 380 degrees F.
Spread the zucchini, potatoes, and red onions in a baking dish. Top with olive oil, tomato puree, and parsley. Season with salt and pepper. Mix all the ingredients to homogenize everything together with the vegetables.
Bake in the preheated oven, stirring after 1 hour until vegetables are tender and moisture has evaporated for about 80 to 90 minutes. Cool slightly before serving.

NUTRITION:
Per Serving: Calories 497 | Protein 9g | Carbohydrates 59g

TOMATO SAUCE

COOKING: 30 min **PREPARATION: 10 min** **SERVES: 6**

INGREDIENTS

- 3 cans of passata
- 1 onion and a half, chopped
- salt to taste
- ⅓ cup fresh basil, torn in half
- 6 garlic cloves, halved
- 3 tablespoons extra-virgin olive oil

DIRECTIONS

In a saucepan, heat olive oil over low heat, then adds garlic and onion. Cook and stir for about 3-5 minutes.

Add salt, passata, and basil.

Cover with lid and cook over low heat, stirring for about 25-30 minutes.

Remove garlic before serving.

NUTRITION:

Per Serving: Calories 152 | Protein 4g | Carbohydrates 20g

THE EASIEST POLENTA RECIPE

COOKING: 15 min **PREPARATION: 5 min** **SERVES: 2**

INGREDIENTS

- 2 cups vegetable broth
- 1/2 cup cornmeal
- 1/2 teaspoon sea salt
- 1/4 teaspoon ground black pepper
- 1/4 teaspoon red pepper flakes, crushed
- 2 tablespoons olive oil

DIRECTIONS

In a medium saucepan, bring the vegetable broth to a boil over medium heat. Now, add the cornmeal, whisking to remove lumps.

Season with black pepper, salt and red pepper.

Reduce the heat. Continue to simmer, whisking periodically, for about 15 minutes, until the mixture has thickened.

Now, pour the olive oil into a saucepan and stir to combine well.

NUTRITION:

Per Serving: Calories: 306 | Protein: 7g | Carbohydrates: 32g

5&1 Meal Plan

WEEK 1

DAYS	FUELING HACKS	LEAN AND GREEN MEAL
1	Tasty Muffins, Breakfast Shake, Fruits Shake Energetic Orange Shake, Fresh Ginger Smoothie	Simple Italian Style Risotto
2	Breakfast Porridge, Cranberry Drink, Amazing, Stawberry Juice, The Perfect Hot Chocolate, Ginger Tea Drink	Vegetables Soup
3	Light Nut and Maple Butter, Lemon Drink, The Detox Ginger Drink, Fabulous Cherry Cider, Fresh Fruit Smoothie	Broccoli Salad
4	Toasted Almonds, The Happy Hour Punch, Classic Mulled Wine, Special Toast, Squash Soup	Spacial Cannellini Beans Recipes
5	The perfect Avocado Dessert, Beans Salad, Fruit Salad, Classic Peanut Butter and Jam Bread, Energetic Ginger Drink	Spicy Hummus
6	Pinapple and Spinach Smoothie, Spinach and Mango Smoothie, Summer Blueberry and Coconut Ice Cream, Healthy Chocolate Mousse, Roasted Almonds with Tamari	The Perfect Quinoa
7	Cinnamon Porridge, Smoked Salmon with Avocado, Easy Hotdog, Blueberry Pancakes, Hot Brownies	Pork Chops

WEEK 2

DAYS	FUELING HACKS	LEAN AND GREEN MEAL
1	Tapas, Iced Mint Tea, Pumpkin Latte, Savoury Oven Pancakes, Shrimp Cocktail	Delicious Roasted Chicken
2	Corn Fritters, Strawberry Smoothie, Cheese Waffles, Vanilla Protein Shake, Tortilla Chips	Glazed Chicken Wings
3	Chocolate Mousse, Indian Crepe, Quick Cookies Snack, Chocolate Chia Pudding, Apples and Almond Porridge	Crunchy Asparagus
4	Homemade Breakfast Cereals, Breakfast Shake, Caramel Penuche, Fresh and Quick Vanilla Ice Cream, Oatmeal and Carrot Cake	Avocado Quinoa Salad
5	Cranberry Drink, "That" Breakfast Porridge, Spicy Coffee, Fruits Shake, The Perfect Hot Chocolate	Quick Cauliflower Salad
6	Honey and Nuts Breakfast, Amazing Strawberry Juice, Ginger Tea Drink, Lemon Drink, The Detox Ginger Drink	Mussel Stew
7	Fabolous Cherry Cider, Delicious Sweet Sandwiches, Savory Muffins, Energetic Orange Shake, Toasted Almonds	Hummus of Cauliflower and Avocado

WEEK 3

DAYS	FUELING HACKS	LEAN AND GREEN MEAL
1	Fruit Salad, Energetic Ginger Drink, Pineapple and Spinach Smoothie, Cabbage and Avocado Smoothie, Roasted Almonds with Tamari	Classic Tofu Stew
2	Cinnamon Porridge, Breakfast Omelette, Quick Zucchini Rolls, Italian Style Omelette, Blueberry Pancakes	The Perfect Quinoa
3	Hot Brownies, Fruit Salad, Iced Mint Tea, Shrimp Cocktail, Strawberry Smoothie	Chicken Meatballs
4	Cheese Waffles, Vanilla Protein Shake, Chocolate Mousse, Quick Cookies Snack, Apples and Almond Porridge	Salad in a Jar
5	Homemade Breakfast Cereals, Cheesecake with Blueberries, Light Nut and Muple Butter, Lemon Drink, The Detox Ginger	Ginger Lime Chicken
6	Fresh and Quick Vanilla Ice Cream, Fresh Ginger Smoothie, Energetic Orange Shake, Amazing Strawberry Juice, Ginger Tea Drink	Tasty Pork with Fake Fried Eggs
7	Savory Muffins, Fresh Fruits Smoothie, Toasted Almonds, The Happy Hour Punch, Carrot Cake	Bacon Mushrooms Dinner

WEEK 4

DAYS	FUELING HACKS	LEAN AND GREEN MEAL
1	Breakfast Wrap, Green Soup, The Perfect Avocado Dessert, Berries Bowl, Energetic Ginger Drink	Bulgur with Spinach and Tomatoes
2	Cabbage and Avocado Smoothie, Healthy Chocolate Mousse, Strawberry Smoothie, Lemon Drink, The Detox Ginger	Patties Kale Salad
3	Tasty Muffins, Breakfast Shake, Fruits Shake, Fabolous Cherry Cider, Energetic Orange Shake	Carrot Fake Meatballs
4	Toasted Almonds, The Happy Hour Punch, Classic Mulled Wine, Special Toast, Squash Soup	Quick Pinto Soup with Herbes
5	Cinnamon Porridge, Delicious Sweet Sandwiches, Savory Muffins, Energetic Orange Shake, Toasted Almonds	Easy Tuna Zoodle Salad
6	Cranberry Drink, "That" Breakfast Porridge, Spicy Coffee, Fruits Shake, The Perfect Hot Chocolate	Salmon with Chives and Scrambled Eggs
7	Toasted Almonds, The Happy Hour Punch, Classic Mulled Wine, Special Toast, Squash Soup	Paprika Chicken with Rutabaga

4&2&1 Meal Plan

WEEK 1

DAYS	FUELING HACKS	SNACKS	LEAN AND GREEN MEAL
1	Breakfast Shake, Energetic Orange Shake, "That" Breakfast Porridge, The Perfect Cereal Breakfast	Tasty Muffin Oatmeal and Carrot Cake	Veggie Risotto
2	Cranberry Drink, Lemon Drink, Fresh Fruit Smoothie, The Detox Ginger Drink	Savory Muffins French Omelette	The Spinach Soup
3	Fabolous Cherry Cider, The Happy Hour Punch, Classic Mulled Wine, Vanilla Protein Shake	Toasted Almonds Sweet Snack Pudding	Broccoli Salad
4	Breakfast Shake, Fruits Shake, Energetic Orange Shake, Fresh Ginger Smoothie	Chocolate Chia Pudding Apples and Almond Porridge	The Easiest Polenta Recipes
5	Vanilla Protein Shake, Strawberry Juice, Lemon Drink, Fuit Shake	Quick Cookies Snack Delicious Sweet Sandwiches	The Curious Coconut Soup
6	Ginger Tea Drink, Iced Mint Tea, The Detox Ginger Drink, Faboulus Cherry Cider	Toasted Almonds Sandwiches	Avocado Soup
7	Fresh Fruit Smoothie, The Happy Hour Punch, Iced Mint Tea, The Ginger Detox	Special Toast Sweet Snack Pudding	Quick Broccoli Rabe

WEEK 2

DAYS	FUELING HACKS	SNACKS	LEAN AND GREEN MEAL
1	The Ginger Detox, Pumpkin Latte, Savoury Oven Pancakes, Shrimp Cocktail	Cheese Waffles Quick Cookies Snack	Classic Hummus
2	Vanilla Protein Shake, Toasted Almonds, The Happy Hour Punch, Strawberry Smoothies	Chocolate Mousse Tasty Muffin	Green Soup
3	Breakfast Shake, Fuit Shake, Cranberry Drink, Energetic Orange Shake	Fresh Mango Cream Fruit Salad	Orzo Salad
4	Spicy Coffe, Ginger Tea Drink, Lemon Drink, The Detox Ginger Drink	Classic Mulled Wine Special Toast	Squash Soup
5	Breakfast Shake, Fruits Shake, Fabolous Cherry Cider, Energetic Orange Shake	Sweet Snack Pudding The Hot Chocolate	Avocado Quinoa Salad
6	Cinnamon Porridge, Smoked Salmon with Avocado, Easy Hotdog, Blueberry Pancakes	Green Olived Toasted Breads Hot Brownies	Protein Chicken with Rice and Tomato
7	Strawberry Smoothie, Iced Mint Tea, Fruits Shake, Fabolous Cherry Cider	Tasty Muffin Oatmeal and Carrot Cake	Hummus with Tomatoes

WEEK 3

DAYS	FUELING HACKS	SNACKS	LEAN AND GREEN MEAL
1	Honey and Nuts Breakfast, Amazing Strawberry Juice, Ginger Tea Drink, Lemon Drink	Light Nut and Maple Butter Classic Avocado Toast	Quick Zucchini Rolls
2	Vanilla Protein Shake, "That" Breakfast Porridge, Spicy Coffee, Fruits Shake	The Perfect Hot Chocolate Savory Muffins	Classic Tofu Stew
3	Cranberry Drink, The Perfect Avocado Dessert, Berries Bowl, Energetic Ginger Drink	Cinnamon Porridge Roasted Chickpea Snack	Cheesy Eggs
4	"That" Breakfast Porridge, Spicy Coffee, Fruits Shake, The Perfect Hot Chocolate	Blueberry Pancakes Tapas	Delicious Roasted Chicken
5	Corn Fritters, Strawberry Smoothie, Cheese Waffles, Vanilla Protein Shake	Rollups with Cheese Cheese Waffles	Lemon Salmon
6	Vanilla Protein Shake, Amazing Strawberry Juice, Fresh Ginger Smoothie, Energetic Orange Shake	Light and Maple Butter Classic Avocado Toast	Crunchy Asparagus
7	Spicy Coffe, Ginger Tea Drink, Iced Mint Tea, Lemon Drink	Savory Muffins Sandwiches	Special Cannellini Beans Recipe

WEEK 4

DAYS	FUELING HACKS	SNACKS	LEAN AND GREEN MEAL
1	The Detox Ginger Drink, Fresh Fruit Smoothie, Fabulous Cherry Cider, The Happy Hour Punch	Sweet Snack Pudding The "Hot" Chocolate	Quinoa Mix
2	Tasty Muffins, Breakfast Shake, Fruits Shake, Fabolous Cherry Cider	Toasted Almonds Sweet Snack Pudding	Vegetables Soup
3	Homemade Breakfast Cereals, Cheesecake with Blueberries, Light Nut and Muple Butter, Lemon Drink	Tasty Muffin Oatmeal and Carrot Cake	Broccoli Salad
4	Fruit Salad, Energetic Ginger Drink, Pineapple and Spinach Smoothie, Cabbage and Avocado Smoothie	Quick Cookies Snack Sweet Snack Pudding	Pork Chops
5	Fruit Salad, Iced Mint Tea, Shrimp Cocktail, Strawberry Smoothie	Hot Brownies Special Toast	Traditional Spanish Tortilla
6	Cranberry Drink, "That" Breakfast Porridge, Spicy Coffee, Fruits Shake	Cheese Waffles Quick Cookies Snack	Spicy Hummus
7	Beans Salad, Fruit Salad, Classic Peanut Butter and Jam Bread, Energetic Ginger Drink	Quick Cookies Snack Delicious Sweet Sandwiches	Paprika Chicken with Rutabaga

KITCHEN CONVERSIONS

1 GALLON	1 QUART	1 PINT	1 CUP	1 OUNCE	1 TBLSP	1 TSP
4 QUARTS	2 PINTS	2 CUPS	16 TBSP	2 TBSP	3 TSP	5 ML
8 PINTS	4 CUPS	16 OUNCES	8 OUNCES	30 ML	1/2 OUNCE	
16 CUPS	32 OUNCES	480 ML	240 ML		15 ML	
128 OUNCES	950 ML					
3.8 LITERS						

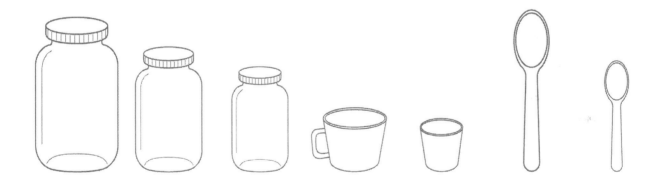

Conclusion

I want to give you a special thank you!

This book is the result of a lot of work and study to guarantee you a cookbook full of tasty and varied recipes. It is a book designed for everyone: those who have little time to cook, those who are always in a hurry, and those who love to cook and spend a lot of time on their dishes.

I hope you can achieve the results you set out to achieve. I want to tell you not to worry if the path seems difficult, sometimes you may think you're failing and feel unmotivated, but I assure you that it's part of the weight loss process and you have to be patient to get the results you want.
Thank you for buying my book.

Made in United States
Orlando, FL
17 June 2022